—— THE ——

PERMACULTURE
KITCHEN

LOVE FOOD

LOVE PEOPLE

LOVE THE PLANET

Carl Legge

Published by
Permanent Publications
Hyden House Ltd
The Sustainability Centre
East Meon
Hampshire GU32 1HR
United Kingdom
Tel: 0844 846 846 4824 (local rate UK only)
        or +44 (0)1730 823 311
Fax: 01730 823 322
Email: enquiries@permaculture.co.uk
Web: www.permanentpublications.co.uk

Distributed in the USA by
Chelsea Green Publishing Company, PO Box 428, White River Junction, VT 05001
www.chelseagreen.com

© 2014 Carl Legge, www.carllegge.com
The right of Carl Legge to be identified as the author of this work has been
asserted by him in accordance with the Copyrights, Designs and Patents Act 1998

Designed by Hayley Harland, www.delectablediary.com
Photographs © Hayley Harland, 2013
Photographs on pages 11 and 175 © Carl Legge, 2013

Index by Amit Prasad, 009amit@gmail.com

Printed in the UK by Cambrian Printers, Aberystwyth

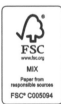

FSC
www.fsc.org
MIX
Paper from
responsible sources
FSC® C005094

All paper from FSC certified mixed sources

The Forest Stewardship Council (FSC) is a non-profit
international organisation established to promote the
responsible management of the world's forests. Products
carrying the FSC label are independently certified to assure
consumers that they come from forests that are managed to
meet the social, economic and ecological needs of present and
future generations.

British Library Cataloguing-in-Publication Data
A catalogue record for this book is available from the British Library
ISBN 978 1 85623 153 4

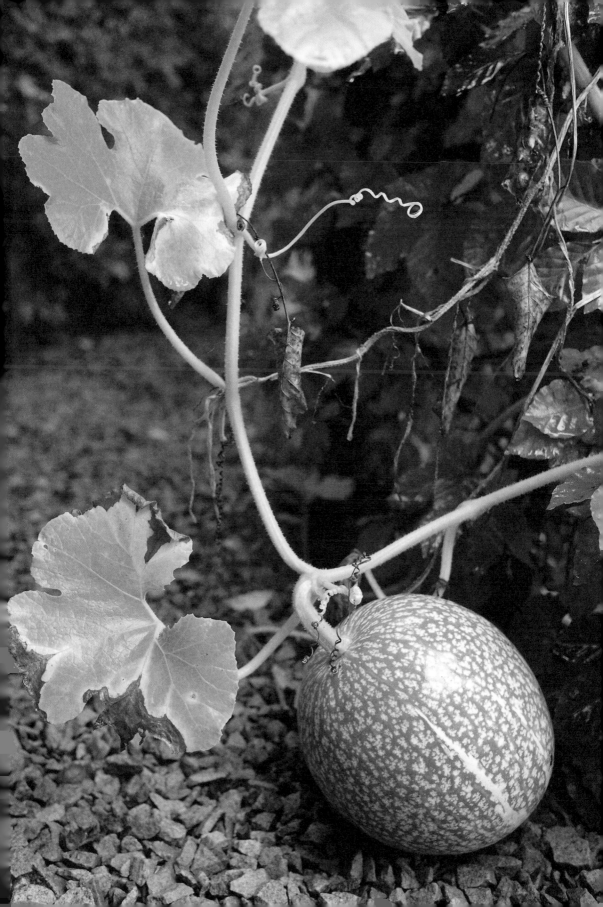

The simple, honest, economy of a kitchen is what turns a house into a place with heart. And that all starts with a good meal that enriches the eater as much as their environment. Carl is a patient and generous teacher and this book teaches us how to make our own recipes as much as it is about following his.

Alys Fowler
Gardener, author and TV presenter

A thought provoking and interesting book, it is structured with basic recipes and building blocks which offer a myriad of variations. There are options that would work for any cook: beginner to competent, vegan to carnivore – not an easy task.

Whilst there is no doubt that this book would be great for someone with a vegetable garden or allotment, here in Central London many of the principles are just as valid. I have no smallholding, but a farmers' market and a hatred of waste unites us.

This is a book to inspire and nourish, one filled with a love of food, family and nature ... one I will return to again and again.

Thane Prince
Author, food writer, cookery tutor
and TV judge on 'Grow, Make, Eat: The Great Allotment Challenge'

I urge you to buy this book, for its simplicity of seasonal life and its complexity in bringing variety in your cooking.

Françoise Murat
Professional landscape designer, teacher of gardening, rural skills and crafts

Here is an inspirational kitchen how-to, by a hands-on gardener and forager for anyone who wants to live sensibly and well, whether you live on a permaculture smallholding or in the heart of a city.

Elisabeth Luard
Trustee Director of The Oxford Symposium on Food & Cookery,
author, journalist, broadcaster

The thinking shopper-baker-cook's handbook for a fun and caring kitchen.

Carla Tomasi
Head chef and owner of Turnaround Cooks cookery school

About the Author 6

Introduction 8

Easy Basics 16

Seasonal Soups 39

Permie Pizzas 58

Creative Curries 64

Quick Veg 86
prepared for pasta, noodles, rice or toast

Grills and Griddles 94

Eggs Are Easy 104

Salads and Dressings 111

Bread is Heaven 136

Preserving Time 151

Tips 160

My Thanks To... 169

Bibliography and further reading 171

Index 172

ABOUT THE AUTHOR

Carl Legge is a self taught cook, forager and home brewer. He may be found wearing camouflage on the Llŷn Peninsula in North Wales. If he's not in the garden growing or picking food, he's in the kitchen cooking it. He lives with his tolerant wife and son on a three-acre permaculture smallholding. Read about Carl's food adventures at www.carllegge.com

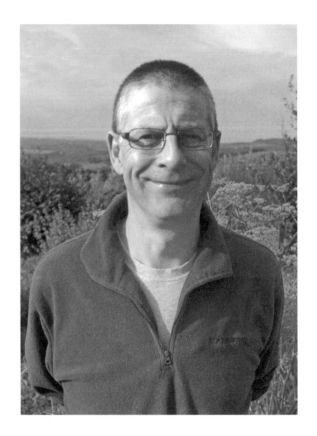

Dedicated to Debs and JJ

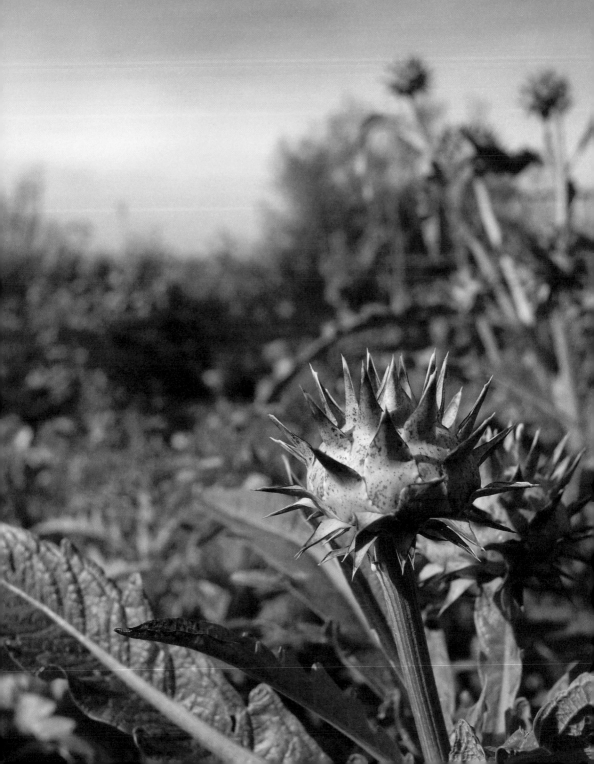

INTRODUCTION

FOOD IS LOVE

The two places in the world where I feel most content and relaxed are my kitchen and my garden. My passion is to grow, prepare, cook and serve fresh, seasonal and great tasting food for family and friends. For me, this is the ultimate expression of love. It's also liberating, creative and enormous fun and I get to drink wine while I'm doing it.

As soon as I had my own places to live in, I grew some of my own food. I've grown herbs and tomatoes in a window in a flat. I took up the lawn in the very small garden of a terraced house and grew mixed fruit and veg.

Since 1997, I have lived with my wife Debs and our son JJ on a three-acre smallholding on the Llŷn Peninsula in North Wales. We're on the side of a mountain overlooking the Irish Sea and Cardigan Bay. It was our dream and our plan to do this and we worked hard to make it a reality. I resigned from a well-paid corporate job to spend time to manage our patch: we swapped money for time. We now grow fruit and vegetables in raised beds, polytunnels and forest garden areas. And we keep chickens because they are fun and provide us with eggs. We've kept pigs, geese, turkeys, ducks and chickens in the past too. What was three acres of subsidised sheep pasture is now a thriving nature reserve, which provides us with a large proportion of our own food.

In my eclectic 'career' I've done some fun 'non-corporate' jobs. I worked in a fish and game mongers cum greengrocers shop. I was the new boy/dogsbody in a bakery. And I had many a happy hour when I worked and tasted my way through various jobs in wine merchants and pubs.

Debs and JJ will tell you that if I'm awake I'm thinking and/or talking about, growing, preparing or eating food. I've cooked now for more than 40 years. I've cooked as a student, a London commuter, a new Dad (with both parents working), a commuter from Wales to London, a government relations consultant and as a busy smallholder/home educator/writer. I write about food to inspire and encourage others to find out how easy and rewarding this cooking lark is.

I've written *The Permaculture Kitchen* to inspire and encourage you to cook sustainably. It shows you how easy it is to cook ethically sourced, seasonal, local food to make tasty meals with no faff, whatever your lifestyle.

The Permaculture Kitchen will help you whether you grow your own, get a vegetable, fish or meat box, or shop at local markets. It will help you answer these questions: "Now I've got it, what do I do with it? How can I make meals with these?"

WHAT'S SPECIAL ABOUT
THE PERMACULTURE KITCHEN?

I know that our smallholding will only help sustain us if we, in our turn, sustain and care for it in the long term. Our contribution is our time, energy and money, which are all limited resources. So we aim to get the best from what we put in. We also try to minimise the things we buy and bring in from outside the holding. And, of course, 'stuff' happens. We see seeds and plants fail and get taken by animals for their own food. The weather is neither reliable nor predictable. We can't always do things outside when we want to. We've had a roof blow off on Christmas Eve and the wind destroy our tall plants. We've seen us and our animals get sick, tired or grouchy. So I don't always have the time, energy or inclination to spend hours planting or cooking, but we must eat to sustain ourselves. If we're not fit and healthy, then we can't manage the smallholding and it can't look after us.

'Permaculture' is a framework of ways to think about, design and manage such a system so all parts are sustainable for the long term. It helps to keep us healthy and happy and to look after our environment and the animals in it. Permaculture principles can be used by anyone, anywhere: city flats; country estates; community spaces; transport systems and commercial and industrial premises to create sustainable systems and places.

In *The Permaculture Kitchen* I aim to help you develop a flexible and intuitive way to cook. The method starts with the ingredients and time that you have to hand and couples those with some foundation principles and basic techniques. The recipes are there to illustrate the principles and techniques. You'll see that I give you ideas for variations of flavours, ingredients and methods. I also give you suggestions for how leftover meals can be used to save you time and energy. In fact, I encourage you to make more than you may need for one meal. This helps you to get some cooking in reserve to save time for when you're pressed later.

With *The Permaculture Kitchen* I help you get connected to the ebb and flow of the seasons, your local climate and weather: more so if you grow or produce your own food. Even if you don't grow your own, you'll have a connection to the providers of your food and their experience of these natural cycles.

The Permaculture Kitchen helps you to get the most from what you have and harvest. You will learn how to make some useful preserves, get multiple meals from an ingredient and maximise the flavour and enjoyment from what you cook.

I've included recipes that you could say were vegan, vegetarian and omnivore. It's easy to eat well, healthily and sustainably with a diet that is principally or exclusively plant based. I've included options and variations that will help you achieve this.

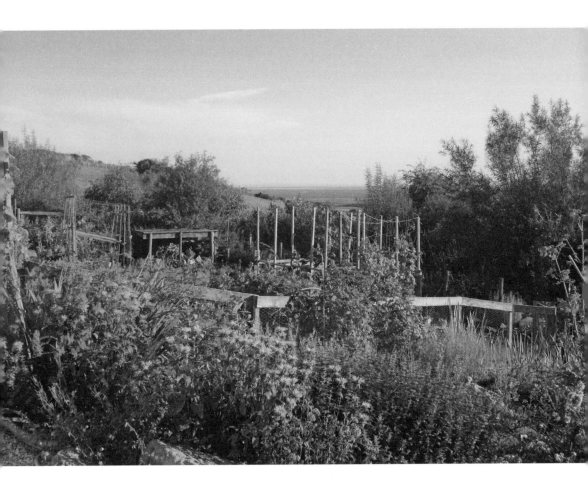

THE PERMACULTURE KITCHEN & SUSTAINABILITY

The Permaculture Kitchen has sustainability at its heart in five ways...

Physical sustainability
The food nourishes you and is tasty and you can prepare it with the tools and equipment you have to hand in the space available in your kitchen. You can cook this food with the minimum of kit in a small kitchen – I do. I'll show you tips and tricks to reduce the time and effort some things take to do.

Temporal sustainability
You can fit how you plan, prepare and consume your food into the time you have available. Sometimes you need a meal that can be on the table in less than 15 minutes. Leftovers, a quick pasta, grill or salad can all be prepared very quickly. When you choose to have more time to cook you can cook something more elaborate or invest in cooking meals to save for later. When you look at your food 'resources' in advance and plan your menus ahead this will liberate you and save time over the week.

Economic sustainability
You can afford the food you use within your budget and your food provider can afford to produce the food you consume. I think that both criteria are important if we're to have vibrant communities and real food. I'll show you how to get the most from your ingredients and to reduce waste. I'll also show you how to use some foraged foods that won't cost a penny to collect.

Spiritual and emotional sustainability
You and your 'audience' appreciate and enjoy the things you cook and how you cook it. This will make you want to maintain the approach. It also means that the whole process is in tune with your collective values. You'll be motivated to continue when you get positive vibes and feel good about what you do.

Environmental sustainability
Your use of food and the treatment of any waste contributes positively to your immediate environment. It also means that your demands on the wider environment are responsible. You'll really notice less waste going out for collection and your bills will be lower.

STEPS IN THE PERMACULTURE KITCHEN APPROACH

I've tried to break down what I do every day and week to cook The Permaculture Kitchen way. It looks terribly organised written down. I promise you once you get into the habit, it feels like a much more organic, continuous process – honest! Once you've got the hang of things, you'll just 'live it' without the need to think too deliberately.

With that in mind here are the three steps in The Permaculture Kitchen approach.

To listen

- To the season and weather.
- To your produce provider: this could be your garden/allotment, your produce box supplier, your market or shop trader.
- To your 'audience', what's their appetite, any special requirements or occasion to cater for?

To survey

- What have I got: from my land or my supplier?
- What's in my larder: basic items and preserved produce.

To design and produce

- So you master basic recipes and techniques for meal construction that help you produce almost everything else.
- A quick 'Guide Menu' for the week to act as a framework for you to plan, shop or harvest.
- Individual meals from example recipes that give suggestions for variations and substitutions.

MENU PLAN

My intention is to produce a menu for the week or the next few days. This helps me to shop efficiently: so I only buy what I'll need to use, it cuts down on waste and reduces the number of trips I make to the shops.

The menu plan is only a guide for me: I often cook something else from what I had planned. What it does is to take away the guesswork if I don't have the inspiration just when I need to start to cook. If you're a member of some sort of box scheme or schemes, it would make sense to plan on the day the most perishable box arrives. This will be the vegetable box if you have the ability to freeze fish or meat.

WEEK'S ACTIVITIES & WEATHER

The first thing I do is put down Debs' and JJ's activities for the week as far as they affect meals. So if Debs is working a late shift, I'll need a meal for us that can be eaten late. Then JJ can have the same if it's cooked in advance or one of the leftover meals from the freezer or cook for himself from the store cupboard. This all helps me decide, for example, whether to cook a meal that will do for multiple days and how to plan to use any leftovers.

I'll often then look at the weather forecast for the coming week, trusting fool that I am. It helps me to decide what sort of dishes might be appropriate to the weather. I get used to disappointment.

INGREDIENTS SURVEY

I then do a physical or virtual survey of my garden, freezer and store cupboard. In the garden, I look for what is ready to harvest and what I have surpluses of. I look to see what I can use to cook now and what needs to be preserved so it does not go to waste. In the freezer, I remind myself what is there and look out for things that may be near to the time that they will reduce in quality.

I'll keep in mind information from the market and shops. I survey what's on offer and talk to the sellers about what is likely to be coming in. I also keep my eye out for end of day bargains and seasonal special offers.

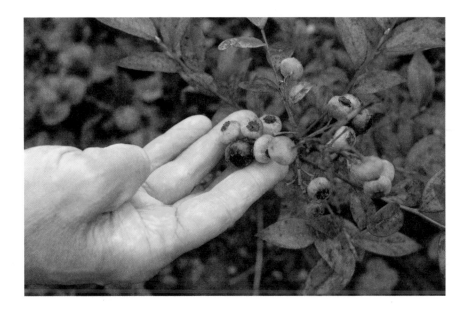

With all that information, I can then plan the week's meals and write my shopping list at the same time. If you do this, it will mean that you will know what to buy so that you don't need to buy things you won't use or preserve for later.

CREATING ATTRACTIVE MEALS

When you design and produce your meals think about how you can meta-phorically and physically 'paint' with your ingredients. Use colours, textures and shapes that make pictures that please your audience's eyes and palates.

ENERGY AND TIME EFFICIENCY

A great way to be efficient with your time and energy when you produce meals is to batch cook. So make up more than you need for the day's meal. Use the extra as leftovers or cool and freeze the surplus in portion sizes. Make sure you label the containers with the date and contents so you know what they are when you go back to them. You will forget otherwise.

In *The Permaculture Kitchen*, all the recipes serve four good appetites unless I tell you otherwise. Please use either the metric measures or the imperial ones: the conversions are approximate and so they don't mix.

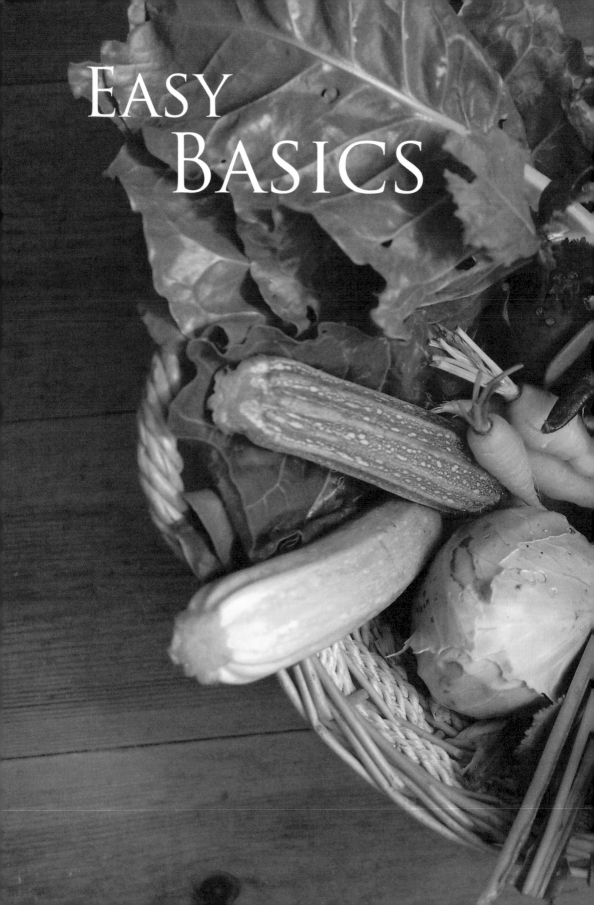

EASY
BASICS

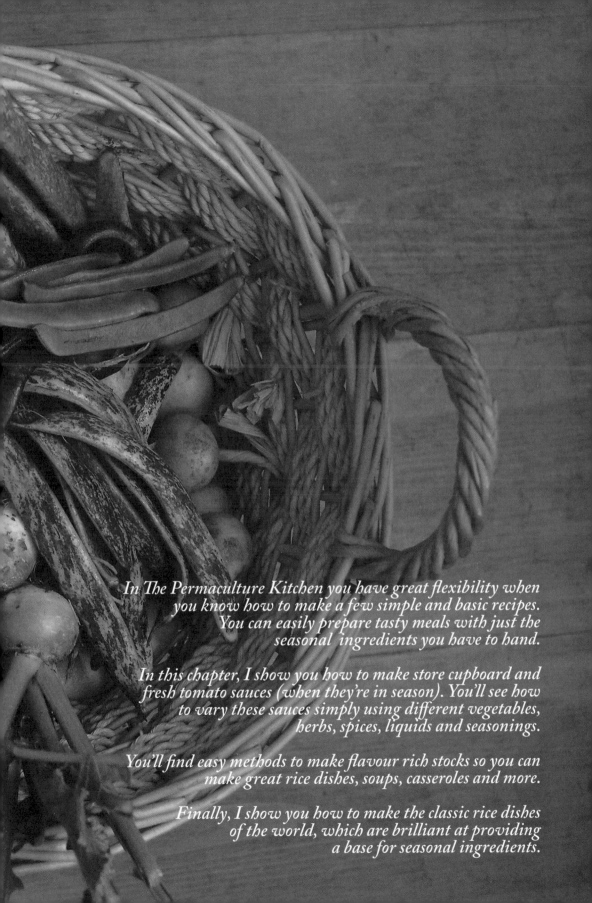

In The Permaculture Kitchen you have great flexibility when you know how to make a few simple and basic recipes. You can easily prepare tasty meals with just the seasonal ingredients you have to hand.

In this chapter, I show you how to make store cupboard and fresh tomato sauces (when they're in season). You'll see how to vary these sauces simply using different vegetables, herbs, spices, liquids and seasonings.

You'll find easy methods to make flavour rich stocks so you can make great rice dishes, soups, casseroles and more.

Finally, I show you how to make the classic rice dishes of the world, which are brilliant at providing a base for seasonal ingredients.

TOMATO SAUCE

The humble tomato sauce is the basis of so many recipes. It may make you think of classic Italian dishes involving pizza and pasta. It's also the basis of many other styles of cuisine from around the world. First, here's how to make the simplest version and I also give you ideas for variations for different occasions.

2 plump cloves of garlic finely sliced or chopped
2tbsp olive oil
1 x 400g (14 oz) tin of chopped tomatoes or
1 x 500g (2 cups) sieved passata
Freshly ground black pepper

The garlic is easier to peel if you first just squash it slightly with the flat of your knife. Not enough to crush it, just enough so it gives. The skin will be looser and easier for you to peel off.

You'll need a wide frying pan or sauté pan to cook this in. The wider the better as you increase the surface area from which the water can evaporate to thicken the sauce.

Warm the pan over a medium heat and add the olive oil. Add the garlic for about a minute until it flavours the oil. Heat gently or you will make the garlic colour too quickly and taste bitter.

Add the tomatoes or passata with a couple of grinds of black pepper and stir.

Simmer gently, stirring occasionally leaving the pan uncovered.

Simmer for about 10 minutes for a pouring sauce for pasta.

Simmer for 30 minutes or more for a thick sauce that will stick to your spatula or spoon and be ideal for a pizza topping. Make sure you keep an eye on this. I've spoilt sauces by wandering away to do something else, allowing them to dry out. Set yourself a timer to make you come back every now and then.

I use this sauce to top my tomato pizzas. It'll make enough to cover a 30cm x 40cm pizza (12 x 16in) or as the base for a pasta sauce for four.

In my house we often eat three quarters of the pizza one night, JJ gets the remaining quarter for lunch the next day and Debs and I have the remaining tomato sauce as part of pasta meal for lunch.

When you simmer away the water, the flavours of the tomatoes intensify. The garlic gently flavours the sauce. Don't add salt as there is often enough in the other ingredients of the recipe you're adding it to. You can season to taste before you serve.

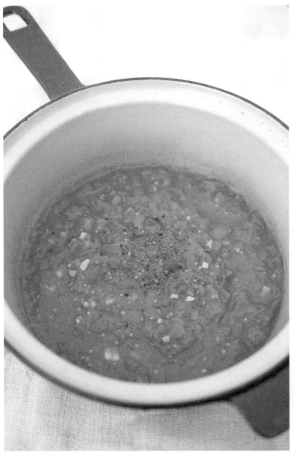
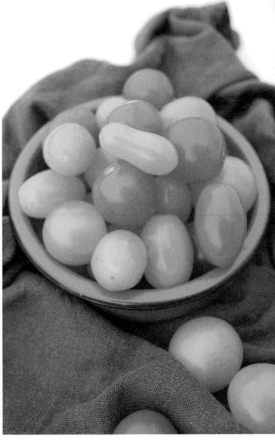

TOMATO SAUCE VARIATIONS

You can of course replace the tinned tomatoes with fresh. If you have access in season to home-grown tomatoes or bought flavourful tomatoes, then this sauce is a delight.

All you have to do is substitute about 500-750g (16-26oz) of fresh tomatoes for the tinned ones. You can skin them and de-seed them, then chop roughly into 5cm (¼in) dice. When I make this sauce with fresh cherry tomatoes, I do not bother to skin and de-seed them.

Add in the same way as the tinned tomatoes. I often put a lid on the pan for the first 10 minutes of the simmer: the liquid is retained and helps the tomatoes break down. After this remove the lid and reduce to your desired consistency.

Plum tomatoes have a higher flesh to water content and fewer seeds than other tomatoes and so make a better 'paste'. This is why they're sometimes called 'paste tomatoes'.

THE CULINARY 'TRINITY': GARLIC, GINGER, CHILLI

When you add the garlic to your sauce, you can also add the other two members of the trinity for an Asian flavour.

The chilli(es) can be added whole, crushed or chopped, using fresh or dry. You'll need to get to know your own chillies so it's best to start with a little and add more.

The chemical that gives chilli its heat is called capsaicin. About 90% of the capsaicin is contained in the white membranes of the chilli that holds the seeds. If you want to manage the heat you can choose to remove or include those parts. Be careful how you handle them and what you do with hands that have touched them. Capsaicin is only soluble in fat/oil so washing your hands with water will not necessarily render you safe. I wash my hands in a little oil and then wash off the oil with soap and water. Also, the capsaicin produces a choking fume if it hits hot oil, so be prepared and keep your cooking space well ventilated.

Fresh ginger is an aromatic root. Depending on the effect you want, you can grate it finely or slice and chop it before you add it to the pan. Finely grate it and the effect will be more subtle. Sometimes you might want to have a bigger texture and burst of flavour than finely chopped or sliced ginger will provide.

If you fry on a high heat, 20-30 seconds cooking will be enough. If you use a medium heat, about 2-3 minutes should provide a nice aroma and flavour.

THE 'OTHER TRINITY': CARROT, ONION, CELERY

This addition to the basic tomato sauce creates a fuller bodied sauce with more complex flavour. This tomato sauce is often used as a base.

Simply chop an onion, carrot and stick of celery into a fine dice and add at the same stage and fry over a gentle heat for 5 minutes before you add the tomatoes. Season to taste with salt and pepper.

'BATTUTO' or 'MIREPOIX'

In Italy and France there is a practice of coarsely or finely chopping onions, other vegetables such as carrots and celery, herbs and sometimes bacon or pancetta. Gently sauté this, covered, as a base for sauces, soups, stews and roasts. Details of this are in the 'Preserving Time' chapter, see page 152.

FRESH & DRIED HERBS

You can use herbs to add flavour to your sauce. As with the garlic, you want to infuse the flavour of the herb into the oil by gentle heating in the initial stage and then add in leaves at the end as a boost of fresh flavour.

With the softer herbs such as basil, coriander and parsley, the best method is to strip the leaves from the stalks. Finely chop the stalks and fry them when you add the garlic to the sauce. Tear or chop the stripped leaves and add them to the sauce when it is finished for a fresh flavour boost.

Tarragon and oregano have harder stems when they are older and so fall between the soft and hard herbs. You'll need to assess what you've picked or bought.

Other, harder herbs can be added with the garlic or onion at the beginning of the fry. The bigger leaves, such as bay and kaffir lime, can be removed if you wish at the end. With thyme, the leaves should be picked and some saved to add at the end. With the rosemary, it can be a bit tough if left whole. I tend to chop it into small pieces before adding.

Dried herbs can be added at any stage.

DIFFERENT SEASONINGS: ANCHOVIES, CAPERS, SMOKED BACON/LARDONS/PANCETTA

I use these ingredients as seasonings. They add a subtle change in flavour to the finished sauce if used carefully.

You can add anchovies with the garlic and allow to gently melt in the heat. Use from a couple of anchovy fillets to 50g (2oz) or more according to the depth of flavour you would like.

With smoked bacon use a small amount, anywhere from 25-120g (1-5oz) or so. You can use bought lardons or pancetta or streaky bacon. How you treat it will depend on the quality of the product you have and how fatty it is. Fry the bacon gently until any water is evaporated. Then continue to fry gently until the fat is rendered out and the bacon is crispy without being burnt. Then you can continue with whatever recipe you have chosen.

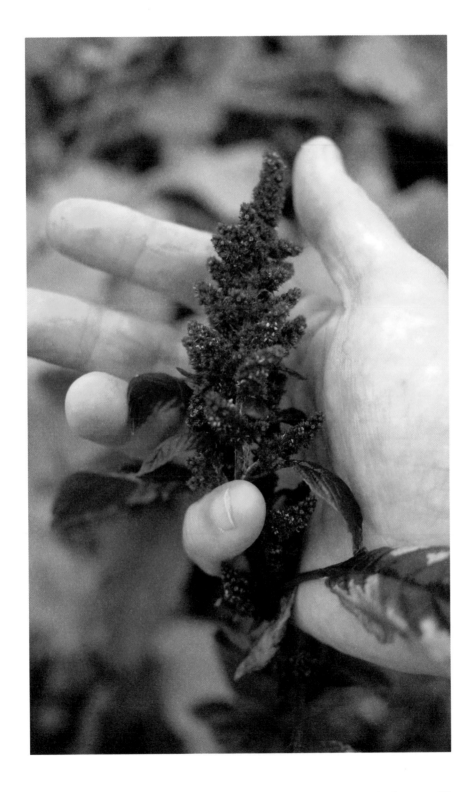

STOCKS

In The Permaculture Kitchen you can greatly improve the flavour of your meal with a well flavoured, home made stock. Use ingredients that would otherwise be thrown away, like leftovers or bones – a great way to get multiple uses from one ingredient. If you don't have the time to make it straight away, then bag, label and freeze your bounty for later.

Sometimes, a stock cube is all you have to hand and is the easiest and quickest option. Look at the ingredients on the pack and buy the best quality you can afford.

For the longer cooked stocks, you can use a pressure cooker to great advantage to save energy and time. When you pressure cook the stock will cloud due to the vigorous, high boiling temperature. This is not a real issue unless you want to make a clear stock for consommé.

I don't put salt in my stocks when they are first made. I have two reasons for this. It's easier for me to control the saltiness if I season the finished dish and if I concentrate or reduce the stock by simmering, the saltiness will increase. So, if you want to put salt in your stock, do this to taste before you serve the dish.

If you want to intensify the flavour of your stocks, just reduce them by boiling once you've strained them.

Your stocks will keep in the fridge for a couple of days. They will keep longer if you freeze or bottle them.

The other quick vegetable 'stock cube' is to use battuto, either made fresh or a frozen chunk cut off a block. See page 152 for how to do this.

The ingredients lists I have given are not prescriptive. All the stocks will have a better flavour if you do use one or more of onion/leek/garlic. So please use what you have that is seasonal or you have stored.

VEGETABLE STOCK

Of all my recipe books, by far the best approach to vegetable stock is taken by Giorgio Locatelli in *Made in Italy*. He advocates using whatever is in season, excluding a few vegetables because their strong flavours would overwhelm everything else. Locatelli's secret ingredient in his vegetable stock is a handful of fresh or frozen peas, which impart a wonderful sweetness to the stock.

I don't use the following vegetables: aubergine; capsicum (sweet pepper); turnips; kohl rabi; brussels sprouts; parsnip; beans; beetroot.

This makes about 2.5 litres (10 cups), so you'll need a saucepan to suit.

2tbsp olive oil
A handful (about 125g/4oz)
of fresh or frozen peas
2 onions
2 carrots
2 sticks celery
2 potatoes
2 courgettes
2 bay leaves
Small bunch of Swiss chard
Small bunch of herb stalks:
parsley/basil/tarragon
6 peppercorns
2+ litres/quarts of water

Roughly chop all the vegetables.

Heat the olive oil in the pan and add the peas. Once they've been heated for a little while, or until soft, mush them up with a wooden spoon or potato masher.

Add the remaining ingredients and cover with water. Bring slowly to the simmer and simmer gently for 20 minutes. Skim if necessary.

Strain the stock. It will not set to a jelly but you can reduce it to concentrate the flavour.

Don't throw away the vegetables. They've released some of their flavour, but are not spent. I freeze what I've used and put them in pie or stew mixes. Not only does it make multiple use of the ingredients, it saves time another day.

CHICKEN STOCK

This will make about 2 litres (2 quarts) of stock. You'll need a fairly big pan somewhere in the range of 5 litres (5 quarts) capacity.

If you want to use an already roasted chicken, pick off the remaining meat from the bones so you can use that in other recipes. If you want to reduce the amount of fat in the recipe, discard the skin.

If you want to use a fresh chicken, check to see if you have giblets inside the cavity and take these out. Pop the giblets, excluding the liver, into your pan. Have another look inside the cavity and remove any lumps of fat.

1 chicken carcass from your roast dinner (or you can use an uncooked whole chicken)
1 onion
2 carrots, scrubbed
2 sticks celery, cleaned
1 leek
2 bay leaves
1 small bunch parsley stalks
6 peppercorns

Pop the chicken into your pan. Depending on the size of your pan, you may need to portion the chicken. Poultry shears or chunky scissors are ideal for this. Use a large bladed knife if you don't have shears or scissors up to the job. Cut down the middle of the chicken through the bone between the two breasts. Then turn the chicken over and cut down or to one side of the spine. You now have two halves. Cut these into portions by cutting diagonally to release the leg portion from the breast portion.

Peel and quarter the onion vertically. Quarter the carrots lengthways too. Roughly chop the celery.

Cut the leeks lengthways in half without cutting the white bulb completely. Fan out the leek and wash away any soil or grit. Roughly chop into large chunks.

Put in your vegetables, herbs and peppercorns.

If you want a deeper colour to your stock, leave the onion skin on; just take off anything that is dirty or damaged.

I cut the veg in this way to increase the surface area exposed to the liquid without making small dice. It means that if I want to quickly strain the stock without using a sieve or colander, I can just put a spatula or skimming spoon across the lip of the pan and keep back the big bits. This saves a bit of time and some washing up.

Next have a look in the roasting pan or container you kept the chicken in. If you've not already used them, you should have some glorious juices left, possibly lovely gelatinous ones. Scoop these into your pan, as they'll add a wonderful depth of flavour to the stock.

Top up your pan with water and bring to a gentle simmer. Simmer for 2-3 hours, skim off any scum that might appear in the initial stages.

If you use a pressure cooker, fill it to the maximum allowed by the manufacturer (mine says no more than half full). Bring the cooker up to pressure and cook for 20-30 minutes and then release the pressure. If you've used raw chicken, you'll need to pressure cook it for about 40 minutes.

Strain the stock and use a fat separating jug if you wish. If I'm in a rush I just put a spatula across the lip of the pan and strain. You can use anything from a coarse colander to muslin to separate out the solids.

If you've used a whole chicken to make your stock, pick off the meat and use in other dishes. It is delicious in pies, pastas, salads or sandwiches.

You can make excellent high quality chicken stock cubes yourself. Reduce the stock to about 25-30% of its original volume. When it cools it should set to a jelly. Pour the stock into ice cube trays or bags before it sets and freeze. When you need some stock you can pop one or more cubes out and dilute them with boiling water. They are also great used neat to 'de-glaze' a pan after a sauté.

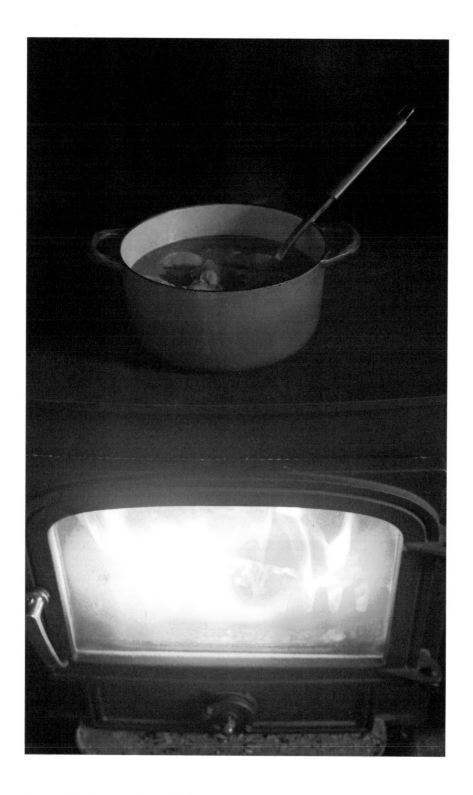

The Permaculture Kitchen

FISH STOCK

You can make the stock with or without herbs.

Wash the fish bones so you get rid of any residual blood, which will cause a scum.

Roughly chop the vegetables.

Add everything to your 5 litre (5 quart) saucepan and just cover with cold water.

Bring slowly to the boil and simmer very gently for 20 minutes. Skim any scum from the surface if necessary. If you simmer for much longer than this you will spoil the delicate flavour.

Strain the stock.

500g-1kg (1-2lbs) fish bones and/or white fish
1 onion
1 celery stalk or fennel bulb
1 bay leaf
Herb stalks: parsley/tarragon/ coriander
6 black peppercorns
1 glass white wine

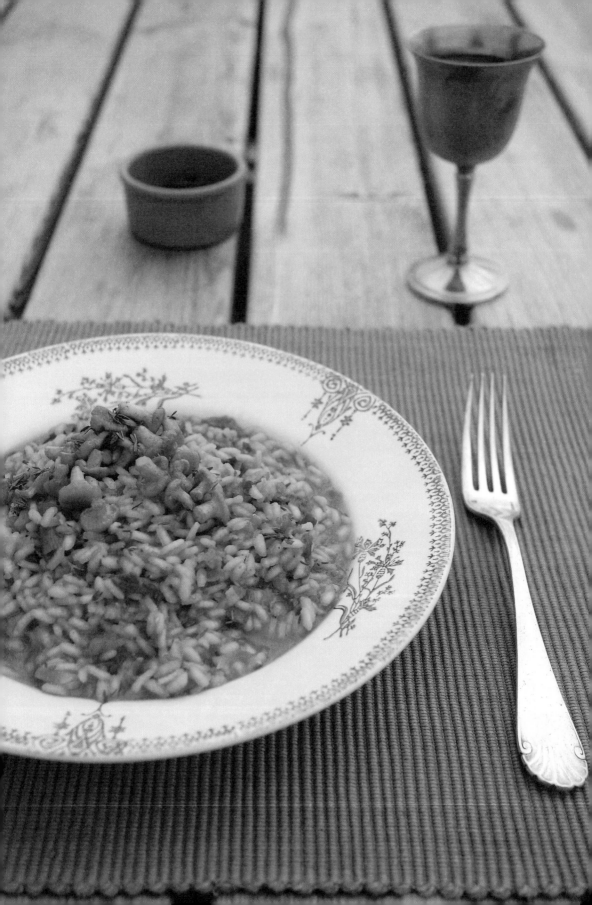

RICE

Pilaf, paella and risotto are just perfect for The Permaculture Kitchen. They are relatively quick recipes, which are at their best when they use fresh, seasonal ingredients. It is a good way to use leftovers or small amounts of veg picked from the garden or left over from other meals. Once you've used the method a few times, you'll easily be able to create fresh meals that satisfy.

Each recipe is a variation on the theme of:

- Fry vegetables
- Add rice
- Add stock
- Simmer

Each cooking method produces different effects. The pilaf is made with high starch long grain rice (I tend to use basmati) and the grains stay separate and distinct. Both risotto and paella are made with medium grain rice with lower starch content. Stir the risotto while it cooks to produce creamy rice with an al dente middle. Do not stir paella continuously as the grains will stay more separate and distinct than in risotto. To produce the peak of paella perfection, allow the grains to lightly toast on the bottom of the pan.

You can vary the taste and texture of each method by using different vegetable, meat, herb and spice accompaniments.

These rice dishes can be meals in themselves as well as accompaniments to other dishes. Leftover rice kept in the fridge is great the next day, eaten cold or converted into other dishes. I'll highlight some uses for the leftovers as you read through.

PILAF

There are as many styles of pilaf as there are names for it. The Permaculture Kitchen method I show you is the most straight forward and useful.

Your choice of oil is very important as it determines a significant part of both the flavour and mouth feel of the finished dish. Butter and ghee both give a much fuller taste and feel than vegetable oils. Vegetable oils let the other ingredients speak more for themselves.

___

3tbsp olive oil, groundnut oil, rape seed oil, butter or ghee
1 large onion, finely chopped
250g (8oz) basmati or other long-grain rice (weighed in a measuring jug so you can check the volume)
Double the volume of rice in hot stock or boiling water
Salt and pepper to taste

A pan with a lid

Warm the oil on a medium heat. Add the finely chopped onion and fry until it is soft and translucent.

Add the rice and fry gently, stirring so that all the grains get coated in the flavoured oil. Fry until the grain begins to change colour and go translucent. Do not brown the rice.

Pour in your hot stock or boiling water. You need twice the volume of the rice.

Return to the boil, cover with a tight fitting lid, turn down the heat to the lowest setting and leave for 15 minutes.

By this time the rice should be perfectly cooked and the grains separate. If you're feeling posh, the rice can be formed into a ring and your chosen meat or vegetables placed in the middle.

Pilaf can be eaten hot, warm or cold. Hold the rice in the pan with the lid on until you are ready. It'll stay warm for quite some time and will not dry out.

PILAF VARIATIONS

Like with the tomato sauce, other vegetables and spices
can be added when the onion is fried or just after.
The rice can be topped in the pan with uncooked
seafood or part or fully cooked pulses or meat.

Leftover pilaf can be used as the filling for pasties,
samosas, or boreks using shortcrust, filo or yoghurt
pastry. It also makes great egg fried rice the next day.

PAELLA

This quintessential Spanish dish has three basic ingredients: rice, saffron and olive oil. It's traditionally cooked in the wide two-handled pan from which it takes its name: the paellera. The pan increases the surface area of the rice touching the bottom to produce the toasted Socarrat. If you don't have a paella pan just use the widest frying pan you have.

Paella has many traditional accompaniments: beans, seafood, chicken, rabbit. Here is the basic method.

3tbsp olive oil
1 onion, finely chopped
3 cloves garlic, finely chopped
500g (1lb) fresh tomatoes, peeled and the skins discarded (you could use strained chopped tinned tomatoes)
1tsp smoked paprika
500g (1lb) paella rice
1tsp saffron
1 litre (1 quart) hot stock

Put the saffron in the hot stock.

Heat the olive oil in your paella pan or substitute. Add the onion, garlic and smoked paprika and fry over a medium heat until the onion and garlic are soft and translucent. Add the tomatoes and simmer for 5 minutes or more until the sauce thickens.

Add the rice, saffron and stock, season to taste and stir to combine the ingredients. Don't stir after this point. Bring to the boil and then cook at a fast simmer uncovered for 5 minutes. Turn down to a gentle simmer for 10 minutes until the stock is fully absorbed.

Then turn up the heat to toast the rice on the bottom of the pan for about 5 minutes. Your ears and nose will tell you when the rice is toasted because it will crackle and smell fragrant. Have a sneaky look with a spoon to make sure it's toasting nicely and you're not burning the rice. Hopefully, the rice should be al dente with a small chalky centre. Take the paella off the heat and cover with foil or a tea towel and allow to rest for another 5-10 minutes. Tuck in!

PAELLA VARIATIONS

Here are some simple ways to jazz it up by incorporating other ingredients.

Big stuff such as boned chicken (leg meat is best), rabbit portions, sausages. Or larger pulses such as butter, fava, haricot and lima beans, chick peas (garbanzos), etc.

Sauté the meats first so they are cooked or nearly cooked through. Then fold them into the rice when you add the stock.

Soak (if necessary) and cook the pulses until they are tender (the pressure cooker is an energy and time saving way to do this). Drain and then tuck them into the rice when you add the stock.

Little stuff such as seafood – prawns, mussels, fish fillets. Or little vegetables – courgette chunks, peas, French beans etc.

Add the seafood in the last 5 minutes fast boil if raw, or in the 5-10 minute covered period if cooked.

Add the little vegetables in the 10 minute simmer if you want them soft, or in the 5 minute fast boil at the end if you want them crunchier.

Leftover paella can be used to stuff sweet peppers or large tomatoes, drizzle with olive oil and bake for 20-30 minutes in a medium oven. If the ingredients match, this is great with grated cheese on top such as manchego or cheddar.

RISOTTO

Risotto is classic Italian cuisine. Your aim is to produce soft and creamy waves of rice with a slight al dente crunch when you bite. You can make risotto simply with only rice and hard cheese or more complex with mixed seafood as well. You can have your risotto to eat in less than 30 minutes. Risotto is fast comfort food.

My friendly Italian food chum on Twitter, Chef Carla, recommends arborio because it releases lots of starch easily to make a dreamy, creamy meal.

This is a recipe for a basic white risotto. It can be used as a starting point, incorporating other ingredients at each stage. With deeply flavoured stock, fragrant wine and the umami of good parmesan, this will be a joyful experience.

1.5 litres (6 cups) stock, kept hot in a pan close to your risotto pan, have a ladle handy
50g (2oz) butter
1 large onion, finely chopped
2-3 garlic cloves, finely chopped
400g (14oz) risotto rice (arborio and carnaroli are widely available)
125ml (½ cup) dry white wine or vermouth
50g (2oz) butter, cut into cubes and chilled
100g (4oz) finely grated hard cheese such as parmesan or pecorino
Salt and pepper

Melt the first 50g (2oz) of butter in a heavy based sauté pan and cook the onion and garlic gently until softened but not coloured (about 5 minutes). If you need to, add a little more butter or olive oil.

Add the rice and stir so that it coats with the flavoured butter and heats through, it will look a little translucent.

Pour over the wine or vermouth, stir, raise the heat and allow the wine to evaporate completely.

Ladle in the warm stock, stirring the mixture constantly over a medium heat. When the liquid is nearly all incorporated, add the next ladleful. Do this for about 10-15 minutes until the rice is soft outside and al dente in the middle. You want the risotto moist (not dry or soupy) at this stage.

It's important to add warm stock so that you do not have to heat it up to temperature in your sauté pan. The result is quicker and better textured. Turn off the heat and cover the pan with a lid. Allow to rest for up to 5 minutes.

Add your chilled butter cubes and hard cheese and beat them into the risotto. Check taste and season appropriately.

RISOTTO VARIATIONS

Before you fry the vegetables, you can add diced smoked bacon, pancetta or prosciutto and fry gently until the fat renders and the meat is slightly crisp.

When you fry the onion and garlic, you can include other flavourful vegetables in the mixture such as finely diced carrot, celery, fennel or stalks of basil or parsley to contribute flavour, texture and colour. If you have made the battuto (see page 152) ahead of time, this is an ideal place to use it instead of the diced vegetables.

At this stage, you can also add sliced fresh chillies, dried chilli flakes, fennel, coriander or cumin seeds. Or you could include meat, such as Italian sausages (sliced or split open and meat removed), that will contribute flavour and requires longer cooking.

Instead of the white wine or vermouth you can add red wine to go with mushrooms, minced beef or cheese. With seafood or smoked seafood, you can use vodka, Pernod or Noilly Prat.

RISOTTO *continued*

After you have toasted the rice and before you add the stock, you can also add: saffron, dried tomatoes, dried mushrooms, other spices such as ground coriander, cumin, cinnamon or paprika.

Additional flavour ingredients can be included during the main cooking of the rice with the stock. These should be either cooked or part cooked so that they just need heating through or finishing off. Choose from:

- Asparagus
- Artichokes, baby ones sautéed, cooked hearts
- Beans, French or runner, blanched
- Beans, such as borlotti, fully cooked
- Cauliflower, in very small florets, blanched
- Courgette, sliced or diced, griddled strips
- Fennel, sautéed
- Garlic, roasted whole cloves
- Nettles, blanched and squeezed dry
- Mushrooms, sautéed
- Peas
- Pumpkin (nice with spices such as cinnamon, nutmeg, cardamom), part-cooked by roasting or poaching
- Seafood (prawns, clams, mussels, langoustine, scallops)
- Woody herbs such as thyme and rosemary

And lastly, you can include other flavour ingredients at the end with the butter. Simply stir through and leave the risotto covered. Choose from:

- Pesto
- Persillade (see page 154 for the recipe)
- Other hard cheeses
- Softer cheeses such as blue cheese, ricotta or mascarpone
- Fried breadcrumbs
- Soft herbs such as basil, mint, coriander, tarragon

The classic use for leftover risotto is to make Sicilian arancini (translated means 'little oranges'). You make them by stuffing balls of the risotto with meat or tomato sauce, or mozzarella cheese; coat them in breadcrumbs and deep fry or bake them. They are wickedly filling.

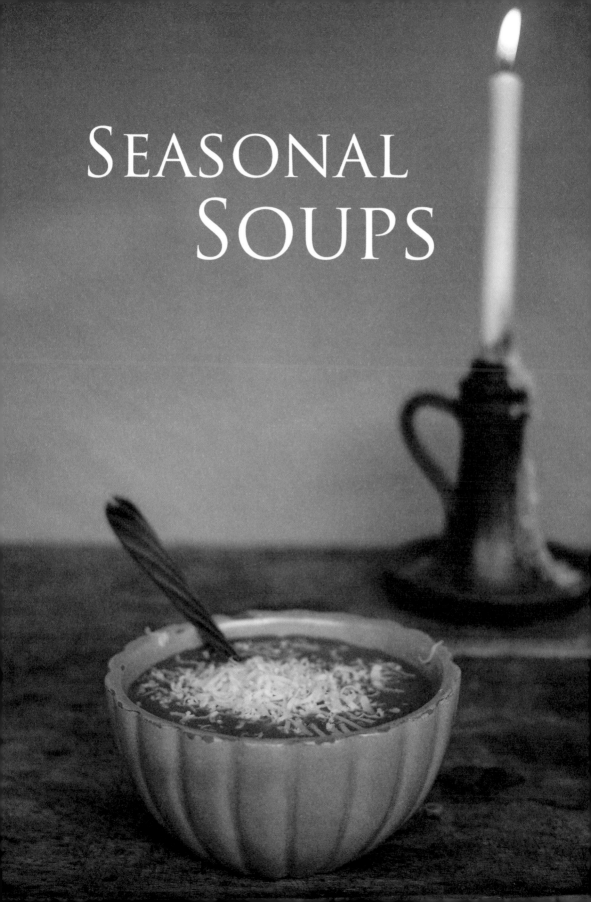

SEASONAL
SOUPS

Here's how to make great soups from simple seasonal ingredients and how to vary the recipes according to what you have available.

It's no surprise that leftover soup sometimes tastes even better the next day. So you may want to make more than you need for just one meal. If you don't eat the leftovers, freeze or can the soup for a meal another day.

LEEK & POTATO SOUP

This is one of my favourite seasonal soups for when the nights draw in and you need comfort food to warm you. It's splendidly easy and a very flexible recipe, which you can play flavour and texture tunes with. You can make a rustic and hearty meal or an elegant dinner party starter.

The key to good soup is the stock. For this recipe, you can use well flavoured vegetable or chicken stocks (see pages 24-27 for recipes).

Make sure you clean the leeks properly. Because of the way they grow, they can accumulate soil between the leaf layers. Unfortunately, when you clean them, it's easy to make them very wet, especially when you pre-slice or chop the leeks first and then rinse multiple times. When you try to sauté them, they will steam or boil. My method to clean leeks gets round this problem because it keeps the leeks as whole as possible. There's less surface area exposed to water and they can be easily dried on a towel. It's not rocket science, but took me a while to suss out.

CLEANING LEEKS EFFECTIVELY

Cut off the leek roots and remove any tough, discoloured or damaged outer leaves. If you are making a rustic soup, keep all the highly flavoured green parts. If not, save them for flavouring stocks and casseroles. Now cut the leek vertically starting a couple of centimetres (¾in) away from the root end so that the leek is divided in two and joined at the root. You can now hold the leek upside down, part and fan out the leek leaves and wash them under running water so all the soil washes away. You may need to give stubborn stains a rub. Then you can dry the leek with a tea towel ready to slice or chop.

Your choice of potatoes and how you prepare them will have a big effect on the soup's texture and flavour. Floury potatoes (like King Edward's or russets) will break down and make a thicker soup. You can control this by the size of dice you prepare. Larger chunks will hold more of their shape, smaller dice will break up. Firm potatoes (like Charlotte or waxy types) will hold their shape and give you a firmer, chunkier finish.

Finally, there is no magic to the precise quantities below. Use what you have and what you fancy. If the soup is too thick, you can always add a bit more stock or water. Experiment and have fun.

1kg (2lb) leeks, washed, as opposite, and roughly sliced
A bunch of parsley, leaves picked and chopped and stalks finely chopped
2 bay leaves, edges torn
2tbsp butter, rapeseed or vegetable oil
500g (1lb) potatoes, scrubbed or peeled and cut into chunks or dice (see above)
1 litre (1 quart) well flavoured vegetable or chicken stock
Salt and freshly ground black pepper

Warm the butter or oil in a large pan over a medium heat.

Add the leeks, parsley stalks and bay leaves to the pan, stir well and cover. Let the leeks sauté over a low heat for 10-15 minutes. They will soften and reduce dramatically in bulk. Keep the heat low so the leeks do not colour.

Add the potatoes and give them a good stir in the leeky/ herby goodness. Pour in the stock and some ground black pepper. Bring to a simmer and cover and cook for about 20 minutes until the potatoes are tender. You could also cook this in a pressure cooker in less than 10 minutes.

Add salt and pepper to taste.
You can leave the soup as it is or adjust the texture. Make it a bit thicker by gently pressing a potato masher through it. Make it smoother by blending with a stick blender or pushing through a mouli.

Garnish with the parsley leaves.

Serve hot with some crusty bread.

LEEK & POTATO SOUP VARIATIONS

Onions/garlic
If you want to increase the intensity of the flavour, you can peel, halve and finely slice an onion or two. Sauté them over a medium heat for 20-30 minutes (or more) so they start to caramelise. Then add the leeks and continue as before.

Of course, you can always add some peeled and sliced garlic to the leeks to contribute a different flavour to the soup.

Other vegetables
Change the flavour and colour of the soup by using other root vegetables in the mix: carrots, celeriac, parsnips etc. If you cut them into fine dice, sauté them with the onions or leeks. If you cut them into chunks, add them with the potatoes.

Bacon
I like to think of smoked streaky bacon as a seasoning. You can also use pancetta, lard fumé or speck. I would add 100-150g (4-5oz) of bacon to this quantity of soup.

Fry the bacon over a low heat so that some of the fat renders and it starts to brown a little. Do this before you add the leeks (or onions). Then add the leeks and continue as before. If using the onions, remove the bacon once it's browned, caramelise the onions and then return the bacon to the pan.

Other meats
This is a great soup to use as a base to use up leftover meats as they will add flavour and substance.

Try shredded or diced roast small game, poultry or pork; or chopped/torn gammon and ham added with the potatoes. Make sure the pieces are bite sized to make eating easier.

Dairy

Traditionally this soup is made with milk or cream. You can replace some of the stock with milk. Just make sure you simmer gently or the milk will curdle.

Alternatively, stir in about 100ml (½ cup) cream or crème fraîche into the soup at the end: then heat gently. Or drizzle an attractive swirl on the top of the soup.

For us, the ultimate comfort food is to have this with some well flavoured cheese grated on top just before we serve.

Herbs

Other herbs that go well in the sauté would be thyme leaves and finely chopped rosemary leaves. Save some of the leaves for the end to garnish.

Chopped chives complement the leek flavour very well: use them as a pretty garnish.

LETTUCE & PEA SOUP

Lettuce and peas are a star pairing for The Permaculture Kitchen. This soup is so tasty and also a top way to use a lettuce glut. It works extremely well with the leaves from plants that are starting to go bitter because they are going to seed. Use green leaves if you want a pure green colour. You can also have fun choosing varieties of different colours.

The peas provide sweetness, so small peas are best. You can also use mangetout and sugar snap peas. Frozen peas of any sort are fine too.

2tbsp of extra virgin olive oil or butter
About 120-150g (4-5oz) of shallots/spring onions/onion finely chopped
500g (1lb) mixed lettuce leaves, washed well and roughly shredded
500g (1lb) peas or similar
800ml (3½ cups) vegetable, chicken or gammon stock
3 sprigs fresh mint, leaves picked (chopped finely if necessary, see right)
Salt and freshly ground black pepper.
Fresh herbs to garnish: see opposite for ideas

Play tunes with the texture of this soup: blend it so it's smooth or leave the vegetables in more rustic chunks. If you do use some of the larger pea pod type vegetables, cut them into bite sized pieces to make the soup easier to sup. And if you're not going to blend it, chop the mint in the recipe finely.

Warm the olive oil or butter in a large pan over a medium heat. Add the shallots or onions and sweat them gently without colouring for 10-15 minutes. They should be soft and translucent.

Add the lettuce and stir in the flavoured oil until it wilts. Pour in the peas, stock and mint. Cover and simmer for 10 minutes or until the peas are tender (this will depend on their size and age).

Check seasoning and add salt and black pepper to taste.

Serve in bowls garnished with fresh herbs.

LETTUCE & PEA SOUP VARIATIONS

Bacon and ham

These have a great affinity with lettuce and peas. Add some (100g/4oz) finely diced smoked streaky bacon, lardons or pancetta to the onions at the beginning. Alternatively, you could put some shredded cooked ham or gammon in with the peas.

Pheasant, rabbit or chicken

Shredded cooked small game or poultry in small pieces adds a meaty twist to this soup. Add bite sized pieces with the peas. If you have some, use fresh tarragon in the soup and as a garnish for a super special taste.

Fish

How about some skinned and cubed white fish poached gently in the soup? You can add, in addition or substitution, some juicy prawns or shelled cooked mussels.

Herbs

Try fresh basil, chives, coriander, dill, parsley or tarragon added to the stock or as a garnish.

Dairy

A swirl of cream, crème fraîche or Greek yoghurt makes a very posh finish for the dish.

Alternatively, beat 100g (4oz) of soft goat's cheese into the soup before you blend it and reheat very gently. If you do this, dill or tarragon are perfect herby partners.

MINESTRONE

In Italian, minestrone literally means 'big soup'. It's The Permaculture Kitchen embodied: a thick, filling soup made from a mix of seasonal ingredients. It's thickened with rice, pasta or potatoes or farro in its many forms. You can use any small or broken up pasta for this.

The taste of your minestrone will depend on the quality of your stock (see pages 24-29) and the quality and freshness of your vegetables. It can be made as a vegan, vegetarian or omnivore meal.

Here are two recipes: one with more spring/summer ingredients and one with more autumn/winter ingredients. Be flexible with the ingredients according to taste and availability.

Paint colours and textures with your ingredients. This list is not prescriptive. The quantities are enough to make a large saucepan's worth (about 4-5 litres/quarts), 6-8 portions depending on appetites.

You can finish off the dish with a rustic dollop of some home made pesto or herb oil preserve (see page 154), or an artistic swirl of spicy olive oil.

Good crusty bread is an essential accompaniment to minestrone in our house.

THE THREE KEYS TO GREAT MINESTRONE FLAVOUR

1. Gently sauté a good vegetable base
2. Use a well flavoured stock
3. Use fresh and seasonal vegetables

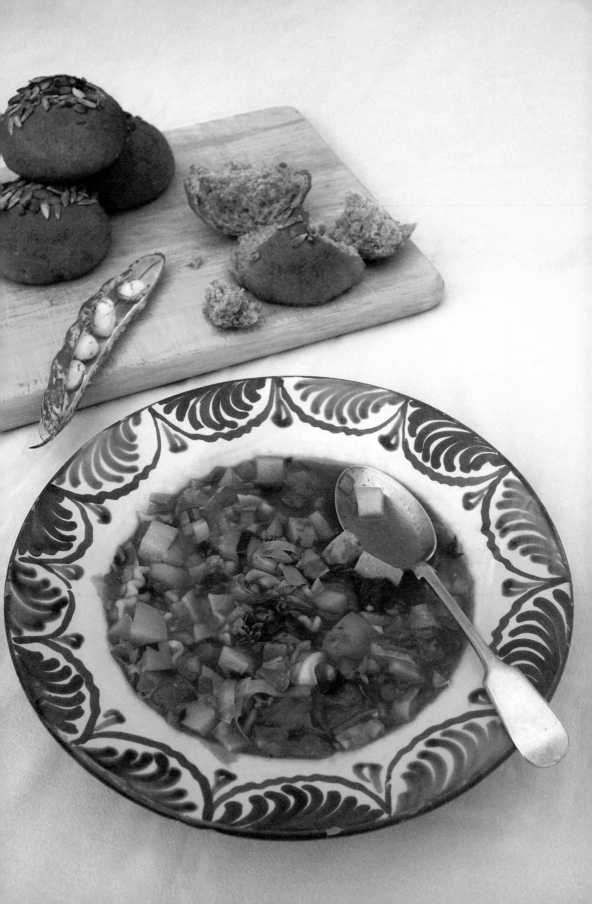

SPRING/SUMMER MINESTRONE

Vegetable base
1 onion, finely chopped
3 cloves garlic, finely chopped
200g (7oz) carrots, finely diced
Small bunch parsley stalks, finely chopped
Small handful of the ribs from chard leaves, chopped
100-150g (4-5oz) of streaky bacon, pancetta or similar, diced (optional)
200g (7oz) baby courgettes, finely diced
3tbsp extra virgin olive oil

Or use a good chunk of your pre-made battuto (see page 152)

Stock
2 litres (2 quarts) fresh stock: vegetable, chicken or ham (if you don't have this to hand or time to make it, use the best quality bouillon cubes or powder you can get or use water).

Soup contents
You'll need 3 or 4 good handfuls of vegetables, remembering that any leaves will cook down.

Baby carrots, halved
Fresh peas (or frozen)
Broad beans
Artichoke hearts, cut into mouthful sized pieces
Small courgettes, chopped in small dice
50-100g (2-4oz) of pasta in pieces
Leaves from the chard above
Lettuce, shredded
Radicchio, shredded
Salt and freshly ground black pepper, to taste

Garnish
Courgette flower petals
Chopped parsley leaves
Extra virgin olive oil or one of pesto, persillade or another of your herb oil preserves (see page 154)
Finely grated hard cheese such as parmesan or pecorino romano or vegetarian equivalents

Pour the olive oil into the pan and heat. Add all the vegetable base ingredients and sauté over a low heat, with the pan covered for 10-15 minutes. You want the ingredients to soften but not colour.

If you are using battuto, just bring up to temperature over a medium heat. Then add the stock and bring to a simmer.

Add the non-leaf contents to the pan, stir well and bring back to the simmer. Simmer for about 10-15 minutes until the vegetables and pasta begin to get tender.

Add the leaves to the pan and stir well. Simmer for another 5 minutes.

Check the consistency of the minestrone and add more stock or water if it's too thick. Check the seasoning and add salt and freshly ground black pepper to taste.

Serve in bowls and decorate with your chosen garnish.

Accompaniments
All this needs is some warm bread to accompany it. Some rustic sourdough (see page 144) or ciabatta would fit nicely.

AUTUMN/WINTER MINESTRONE

Beans

200g (7oz) of fresh beans such as borlotti or haricot or dried beans soaked for a
minimum of 4 hours (see box on page 52 for guide to cooking beans)
1 bay leaf, edges torn
Or, use a 400g (14oz) tin of beans, drained and rinsed very well
Salt and freshly ground pepper, to taste
Extra virgin olive oil

Vegetable base

1 onion or leek, finely chopped
3 cloves garlic, finely chopped
200g (7oz) carrots, finely diced
2 sticks celery, finely chopped
½ -1 bulb fennel, finely chopped
Small bunch basil or parsley stalks, finely chopped
100-150g (4-5oz) of streaky bacon, pancetta or similar diced (optional)
3tbsp extra virgin olive oil

Or use a good chunk of your pre-made battuto (see page 152).

Stock

1 litre (1 quart) fresh stock: vegetable, chicken or ham (if you don't have this
to hand or time to make it, use the best quality bouillon cubes or powder
you can get)
2 x 400g (14oz) tins of chopped tomatoes; or 1kg (2lb) fresh tomatoes peeled,
de-seeded and chopped, or 1 litre (1 quart) passata
A large glass of red wine

Soup contents

You'll need 3 or 4 good handfuls of vegetables, remembering that any leaves will
cook down.

Baby carrots, halved
Courgettes, chopped in small dice
Root vegetables, diced (turnips, swede, potato, salsify, kohl rabi)
50-100g (2-4oz) of pasta in pieces
Kale, shredded

Cabbage, shredded
Spinach, shredded
Salt and freshly ground black pepper, to taste

Garnish
Courgette flower petals
Basil leaves
Extra virgin olive oil or one of pesto, persillade or another of your herb oil preserves (see page 154)
Finely grated hard cheese such as parmesan or pecorino romano

Pour the olive oil into the pan and heat. Add all the vegetable base ingredients and sauté over a low heat, with the pan covered for 10-15 minutes. You want the ingredients to soften but not colour. If you are using battuto, just bring up to temperature over a medium heat and fry gently, covered.

Then add the stock, tomatoes and wine and bring to a simmer for 15 minutes to thicken and allow the flavour to become smoother.

Tip the non-leaf soup contents into the pan, stir well and bring back to the simmer. Simmer for about 10-15 minutes until the vegetables and pasta are just starting to get tender.

Add the leaves to the pan and stir well. Simmer for another 5 minutes.

Check the consistency of the minestrone and add more stock or water if it's too thick. Check the seasoning and add salt and freshly ground black pepper to taste.

Serve in bowls and decorate with your chosen garnish.

Accompaniments
All this needs is some good bread to accompany it. Some rustic sourdough (see page 144) or ciabatta would fit nicely.

HOW TO COOK DRIED BEANS

You need to cook the beans separately. There is a lot of dodgy information about cooking beans. Some of it from famous chefs is plain wrong. If you cook beans in acidic water they will not soften. It's why part-cooked kidney beans never get any softer in chilli sauce; the tomatoes make the sauce acidic. Here's how to cook them so they are tender.

Soak them overnight in cold water, or for a few hours in water that has just boiled. They will be hydrated when their wet weight is about twice their dry weight. Then drain and rinse them.

Put your beans in a pan with a bay leaf and cover with water. If you use boiling water, the outside can go mushy before the inside is cooked. So if you have time, use cold water and bring to a simmer. Cover and check for tenderness and water coverage regularly so that the beans do not dry out. Fresh beans may take 20 minutes or so, dry beans from 40 minutes upwards depending on how old they are. The beans will take less than 10 minutes to cook in a pressure cooker. I often save the cooking water to use as a stock.

Once the beans are tender, drain them and season them lightly with salt, pepper and olive oil.

FISH CHOWDER

This is a fish soup thickened with potatoes. You can play culinary tunes when you use seasonal ingredients.

In line with The Permaculture Kitchen approach of 'painting with food', you can use a mixture of different fish (e.g. salmon, smoked haddock, pollock: pink, light gold, white). Different coloured vegetables also work very well here. So the recipe is ideal for using up little amounts of food that otherwise might go to waste.

The word chowder is thought to originate from the French word chaudière (boiler or pot). In the 18th century Breton fishermen took the idea of this thick fish soup (called Cotriade) to the Newfoundland fisheries. Tragically, the fisheries collapsed in the early 1990s because they were over fished, so make sure that whatever fish you use is from sustainable sources.

In a large pan warm the oil or fat over a medium heat. Add bacon if using and fry gently until it has rendered some of its fat and starts to brown.

Then add the onions/leeks, chopped herb stalks and bay leaves and sauté them all gently until tender and fragrant. Do not allow them to colour.

Add the potatoes and quickly stir round in the fragrant oil and vegetables, then pour in the stock. Bring to the boil and simmer, cover for about 10 minutes until the potatoes are just becoming tender. The actual timing for this will depend on the variety of potato and how small you cut them – smaller chunks cook more quickly.

1-2tbsp olive oil (or use lard or butter)
50-100g (2-4oz) smoked streaky bacon, pancetta or similar, finely chopped (optional)
1 onion chopped and/or
2 medium leeks, split, washed, dried and sliced
Bunch of fresh herbs, leaves picked and soft stalks chopped finely
3 bay leaves, edges torn
500g (1lb) potatoes, scrubbed or peeled and cut into chunks or dice
1 litre (1 quart) fresh stock (use well flavoured fish or vegetable stock, see page 25, 29 or the corn cob stock on page 166)
300g (10oz) fresh fish, skinned and pin boned and cut into mouth sized chunks
Salt and freshly ground black pepper

FISH CHOWDER *continued*

At this stage you can crush the potatoes gently with a masher, spoon or fork to help thicken the soup. Make sure you are happy with the texture now because you don't really want to mess with the soup once the fish is in it.

Add half of the herb leaves and the fish to the potato mix. Poach the fish on the lowest possible heat for 5-10 minutes until it is just cooked through and flakes easily.

Season to taste and serve in bowls garnished with the remaining herb leaves.

Accompaniments
Any hearty bread is great with this, so a sourdough or soda bread would be ideal (see page 144). With the original Breton recipe, Cotriade, the broth was poured over bread to eat first and then the fish and potatoes were eaten separately.

FISH CHOWDER VARIATIONS

Aromatics
In addition to the onion and/or leeks you can use sliced or crushed garlic.

Root vegetables and celery
Add diced carrots, celery and/or fennel to the onion sauté at the beginning. If you have time, a longer, covered sauté over a low heat will help to develop a really deep flavour.

Substitute different root vegetables to the potato for colour and taste variations. Diced carrot, celeriac, kohl rabi, oca, mashua or parsnips would all be good.

Squashes and cucurbits
Squashes and some cucurbits work well. Add diced butternut squash or pumpkin at the same time or instead of the potatoes. Courgettes are best added with the fish.

Herbs

The following herbs will work well: anise, bay leaves, chervil, chives, coriander, dill, fennel, lovage, marjoram, parsley, smallage (wild celery), tarragon and thyme. Make use of the soft stemmed herbs by chopping the stems finely to add with the vegetables when you sauté them.

Spices

The following spices can be added whole when you sauté the vegetables: anise, chilli, cumin, coriander, dill, fennel, saffron, and star anise. Or you could add them in ground form just before you add the potatoes. They give a slightly Mediterranean or south-east Asian feel to the dish. Be gentle with how much you use though, so that the taste of the fish still shines through.

Seafood

Any fish would work with this. In the traditional Breton Cotriade, the fishing vessel's crew would be given the cheaper cuts of fish and these would be used. *Larousse Gastronomique* cautions against using more than 25% of oily fish such as sardine or mackerel. I prefer not to include these fish because their taste overpowers the dish.

Shellfish

Also good to add at the end are prawns, mussels, cockles or clams. Don't use anything that's been preserved in vinegar though.

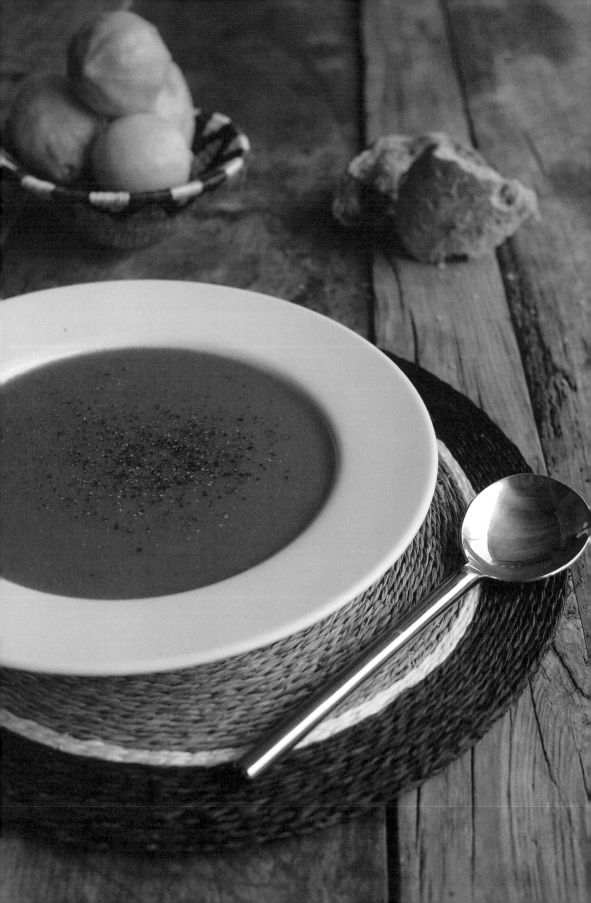

Tomatoes

There's a bit of a tradition that says you should not add tomatoes to a New England clam chowder. If you're not a New Englander and/or not using clams, I think it works well! You can add some roughly chopped fresh tomatoes, once the onion has sautéed and before the potatoes are added, and reduce them down. If you do this, the potatoes may stay firmer as the acid in the tomatoes means the surface doesn't go so soft.

Alternatively add a can of quality chopped tomatoes to the soup with the fish and bring back to a simmer.

Stock and liquid

You can add or replace some of the stock with wine (red or white), vermouth, vodka or vinegar. In all these cases, I'd add them once you've finished the sauté and reduce over a high heat to get rid of any harsh flavours.

Dairy

Dairy products are traditionally added to chowder. You can use milk, crème fraîche, single/double cream or yoghurt. With the lower fat products you need to heat them gently so they do not boil or they may curdle. For added flavour you can steep a clove studded onion, bay leaves etc. in hot milk or cream. Then discard the onion, herb and spice.

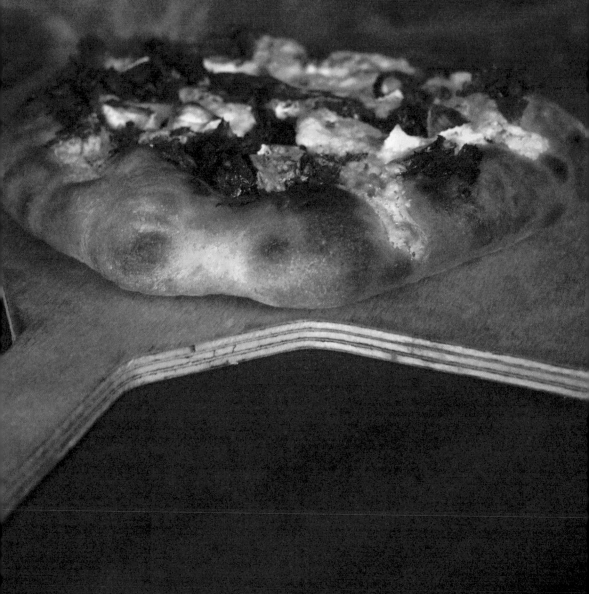

PERMIE
PIZZAS

When you've got the hang of making the pizza base, which is simplicity itself (see page 150), you open the door to the fun world of pizzas. Once in the oven, they cook in a matter of 10-15 minutes or so. Pizzas are so delicious when you use simple, seasonal ingredients and make the most of their texture and flavour.

Pizzas are an ideal way to use up leftovers from previous meals. Slow roast pork can be shredded, extra tomato sauce can be spread. Pizza is brilliant as a quick meal or snack the next day if you haven't eaten all you made.

They don't all require tomato sauce to be made, but as you can see (page 18) that's very easy to make with fresh or tinned tomatoes.

I'm not a huge fan of 'big pizzas': ones with loads of toppings. This is partly because I think the flavours get confused; I call it 'dustbin cooking'. Too much topping can also make the base difficult to cook through quickly and so it ends up soggy.

All the quantities here make a pizza that's about 30 x 40cm (12 x 16in) with a cooked base that is just less than 1cm (½in) thick. I always make the biggest pizza that can fit in my oven. If you're making smaller pizzas, just scale down the ingredients. This quantity would also make two 28cm (11in) or four 18cm (7in) diameter round pizzas.

I cook my pizza on a granite baking stone that really gives a crisp bottom. A pre-heated pizza stone or oven tray, or even using heatproof quarry tiles will also help with this. I make my pizza on Bake-o-Glide™ and transfer this to the stone with a wooden 'peel'. You can make up the pizza on lightly oiled kitchen foil or floured baking parchment and then transfer this on to hot trays to get a crisp bottom.

To make the pizzas, you'll need to have a pre-heated oven: the hotter the better. My oven goes up to 250°C (480°F) and that works fine. If you can't get your oven this hot, don't worry; just give the pizza a bit longer to cook.

FORAGED GREEN PIZZA

2 to 4 big handfuls of foraged greens, for example, nettles (use gloves), bittercress, wild rocket), well washed, drained and squeezed and patted dry in a tea towel
Salt and freshly ground black pepper, to taste

Optional seasonings (choose one or more)
freshly grated nutmeg, chilli flakes, dried oregano, finely chopped garlic

Optional coatings (choose one)
crème fraîche, double cream, extra virgin olive oil

Cheeses
choose from one or more well flavoured, melty cheeses and your local or vegetarian equivalents of these: taleggio, brie, camembert, blue cheeses. Cut them into 1-2cm (½-¾in) dice or random chunks

We love this pizza. As the seasons change you can use different foraged wild greens. Taste the seasons' changes through your pizza. It's dead easy to put together.

The greens will really cook down; so don't worry about the quantity being too much. Some cook down more than others so experiment and have fun.

Lay your greens in a bowl and season well with salt and pepper.

Decide your optional seasonings and sprinkle these in the bowl. Then decide which coating you want to use and add this so the greens are just moistened but not drowned.

Thoroughly combine the seasonings and coatings together with your hands, tongs or salad servers.

Roll or press out the dough to your desired size on the baking sheet, foil etc. Take it steady doing this. If you find that the dough springs back or starts to tear, leave it for a few minutes to rest and then come back to it. You need to persuade it into place, not force it.

Evenly dot your cheese cubes over the dough.

Pile your greens evenly over the cheese.

Pop into your hot oven for 5-15 minutes until the dough is golden and crisp on the edges, the greens have wilted and the cheese has melted and started to brown.

COURGETTE PIZZA

For large parts of late spring and summer these fruits are plentiful. If you are lucky, you'll have access to courgettes with different shapes, textures and colours. So you really can use The Permaculture Kitchen approach to paint a picture on your pizza.

This pizza is another very quick and easy recipe with a fresh taste.

500g (1lb) young courgettes, preferably, mixed colours and textures, cleaned
1-4 garlic cloves (according to taste), peeled and thinly sliced
1 small red onion or 6 spring onions, finely sliced
Extra virgin olive oil
1-2tsp dried oregano
2-3tbsp of persillade, rocket pesto or similar (see page 154 for recipes)

Optional
some parmesan, pecorino romano or equivalent hard cheese, finely grated.

Top and tail the courgettes. Slice them lengthways into approximately 3mm (⅛in) strips.

Roll or press out the dough to your desired size on your baking sheet, foil etc. Take it steady doing this. If you find that the dough springs back or starts to tear, leave it for a few minutes to rest and come back to it. You need to persuade it into place, not force it.

Spread the persillade, pesto or similar over the dough in a thin layer. You are after a thin coat to give a taste, not a complete layer. Gaps are ok, yes really!

Heat a good lug of olive oil in a pan over a medium heat. Put the onion in the pan and sauté for 2-3 minutes. Add the courgettes, garlic and oregano and sauté for another 2-3 minutes to just take the firmness off the courgettes.

Spread the courgette mix straight from the pan evenly over the herbed pizza base. No need to flatten it down, the high spots will brown nicely. Season to taste with salt and pepper. If you fancy, drizzle over a little more olive oil and grate over some hard cheese.

Pop into your hot oven for 5-15 minutes until the dough is golden and crisp on the edges and the courgettes have taken on some colour.

CHEESE & TOMATO PIZZA

Cooked simply, with fresh top quality ingredients, this timeless classic is what most people think of as pizza.

It can be varied with some seasonal ingredients or some classy seasonings. Please don't overdo it, simplicity is best.

About half a quantity of basic tomato sauce made with fresh or tinned tomatoes (see page 18) or just use fresh cherry tomatoes roughly chopped
250g (8oz) good quality mozzarella or local or vegetarian equivalent
1tbsp dried oregano
Extra virgin olive oil
Salt and freshly ground black pepper

Roll or press out the dough to your desired size on a baking sheet, foil etc. Take it steady doing this. If you find that the dough springs back or starts to tear, leave it for a few minutes to rest and come back to it. You need to persuade it into place, not force it.

Spread some of the tomato sauce on to the dough. I prefer to have a thin coat and leave 1cm (½in) or so around the edge of the dough free of sauce. On the rest of the dough the sauce is translucent. If you lather too thick a layer on, the dough will get soggy.

With the cheese, I normally break it by hand into roughly 2.5cm (1in) dice and place it evenly over the tomato sauce. Sprinkle over the oregano and drizzle over a little olive oil. Season to taste with salt and pepper.

Pop into your hot oven for 5-15 minutes until the dough is golden and crisp around the edges and the cheese is melted and slightly browned.

CHEESE & TOMATO PIZZA VARIATIONS

Cheeses

There are a wide variety of cheeses that would go nicely on top of the pizza. Experiment with local cheeses to see what takes your fancy.

SEASONINGS

I count a few things as 'seasonings' for this purpose. The idea is that you use a little of one or two of them to subtly alter the taste of the basic pizza.

- Very thinly sliced red onion, separated into rings
- Olives: either whole or pitted olives halved or sliced
- Roughly chopped capers or pickled nasturtiums
- Anchovies
- Rocket leaves
- Basil or tarragon leaves (I find these can lose their flavour in the intense heat of the oven and so tend to garnish with them once the pizza is cooked)
- Torn prosciutto or pancetta loosely placed on top so edges are exposed and they brown and crisp

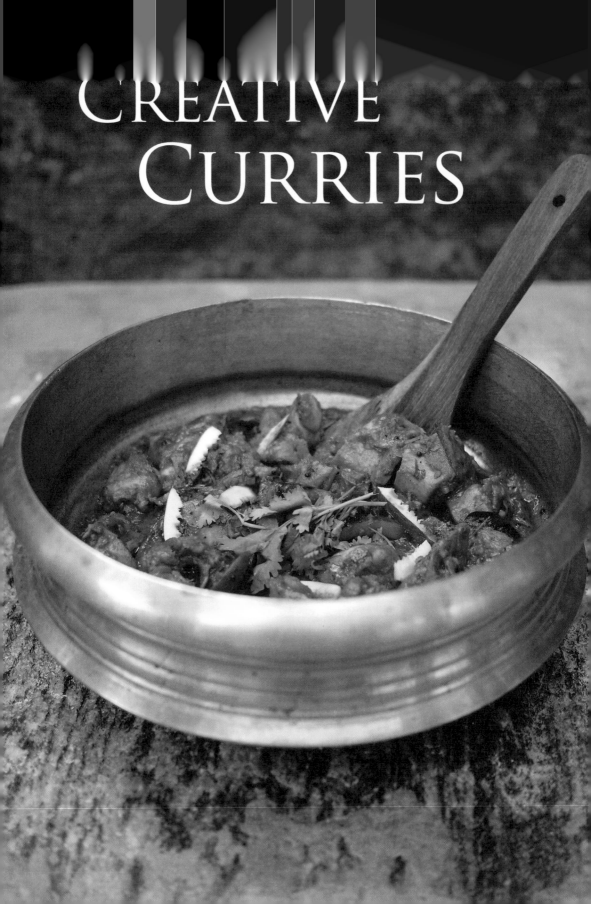

CREATIVE
CURRIES

Curry is a very versatile dish that contains fresh, seasonal produce. You'll find a myriad of ways to make them if you consult the recipe books. I've developed two easy methods to help you start your curry sauce. The first method is similar to the one for tomato sauces and rice dishes where you use chopped vegetables. The second one starts with a vegetable paste.

Once you've got the hang of the basic methods you can use them to make curries with just about anything. I've given you a recipe each for vegetable, fish, beef, and chicken curries. You can then go on to use what you have to hand.

I like to think of curries being fragrant rather than spicy so they stimulate the palate rather than strip it. If you are not familiar with using spices, try the mixes I've suggested. They include some classic combinations. After that sniff and experiment with other spices and mixes. In my view, less is more on the spice front. Mixes of five or more spices often end up in the culinary equivalent of the muddy hues that artists can create if they mix too many colours together. That's not always the case but just remember: more isn't necessarily better. You can use the spices whole or ground.

I don't think that 'hotter curry is better curry'. If your only experience of a meal is the intense burn of chilli, that's a waste of good ingredients and time. My recommendation is to add enough chilli to provide flavour (and different varieties do have different flavours) without burning everything else out. I don't put quantities of chilli in the recipes. There's really little point because of the variability of heat/flavour. Get to know the characteristics of the chillies you use and experiment with different varieties.

I've included a recipe for chilli oil on page 158. If you feel at the end of your cooking that your dish needs an extra kick you can use some of this or let your audience add to taste.

I use mostly peanut oil (groundnut) when I cook curries. It has a nice flavour and a high smoke point which means it doesn't go bitter with high heat. I also use plain vegetable oil or rapeseed oil. I occasionally use the saturated fats ghee or clarified butter for their flavour.

FOOLPROOF CURRY METHOD

Oil (the quantity you'll need will vary depending on the variations you use and these are explained below)
1 or 2 onions
2 or 3 garlic cloves (or quantity to taste)
20g (¾oz) knob of ginger

Optional
Whole spices such as mustard, cumin, coriander *or* cardamom seeds, cinnamon sticks
Ground spices
Fresh or dried chillies, whole *or* chopped, ground cayenne pepper
Meat or other protein (tofu, pulses) of your choice
Tinned or fresh tomatoes
Stock
Coriander or other herbs to garnish

Cook in a deep sauté pan or a saucepan.

If you want to use meat or tofu, allow it to reach room temperature. Cut to your desired size and pat dry. Heat 2 tablespoons of oil in the pan and fry the meat / tofu over a medium-high heat until brown on all sides. Don't try to brown a whole panfull at once. Too many pieces mean that the pan loses heat and there is more likelihood that the meat will ooze liquid and steam. Take out the meat/tofu and put to one side.

If you are using whole spices, fry one or two of them in a tablespoon of oil over a medium-high heat for 1-2 minutes until they are fragrant and the seeds pop. Then continue with one of the variations below.

Variation 1: chopped vegetables
Chop the onion(s) finely. Grate or finely chop the garlic and ginger. Fry the onion, garlic and ginger over a medium-high heat in the oil with the whole seeds until the onion is lightly coloured. You could also add coriander or basil stalks at this stage.

Variation 2: vegetable paste

You'll need a food processor or blender. Cut the vegetables into rough chunks just so the food processor or blender can cope with them. Fresh or dried chillies can be added here too, as can the stalks of coriander, parsley or basil.

Add all the vegetables, chilli(es) and herbs to your machine and process until you have a paste. You may need to add 2 or 3 tablespoons of water to assist the process.

Fry the paste in 2 tablespoons of oil. Be careful because the liquid will spit in the hot oil. Also, the chilli may make you cough a bit as it fries. Stir-fry for 5 minutes or so over a medium heat until the water has evaporated and the paste has a light brown colouring.

That's the variations; you can now proceed the same way for either method.

...continuation for both curry methods

Add the ground spices and stir-fry over a medium heat for 1-2 minutes until they are fragrant.

Add back your meat and whole spices and/or your tofu or pulses. (If you are using dried pulses, do not add salt at this stage because the salt may toughen the pulses.) Stir so that all is well coated in your fragrant vegetable mix.

Now you can add tomatoes and/or stock to your desired consistency and simmer until the meat/tofu/pulses are cooked.

Stir through some chopped herbs and garnish with the rest.

Now that couldn't really be simpler, could it? You can have curry on the table that tastes just great in less than 30 minutes.

DELICIOUS DHAL

This is such a versatile dish. You can serve it as a main meal curry with vegetables or salad. I make lots and keep some for impromptu snacks and energy boosts. It's great scooped up with roti (see page 138) and topped with yoghurt. Or make it really thick and put in sandwiches and wraps with herbs and spring onions. In fact, if you are eating no other protein with your meal, the enzymes in the breads help to make the dhal protein better available to your body.

I suggest two types of dhal to use. You can use what others you have to hand. Split red lentils are a bonus because they do not need soaking. I cook my pulses in a pressure cooker because it's much quicker and uses less energy. Cooking in a saucepan will take longer and you'll need to keep an eye on them and their water level.

Pulse paste
250g (8oz) chana dhal
250g (8oz) moong dhal
1 onion, peeled and roughly chopped
1 carrot, scrubbed and roughly chopped
1tsp ground turmeric
1tsp ground paprika
1tbsp vegetable oil

This quantity will make plenty so you have leftovers to use.

To finish
2tbsp vegetable oil
1-2tsp cumin seeds or panch poron
1 onion, peeled and finely chopped
2-3 cloves garlic, grated or crushed to a paste
20g (¾oz) root ginger, peeled and grated or finely chopped
1 chilli, finely chopped or crushed dried chillies (optional and to taste/heat)
1tsp turmeric
2tsp ground coriander
400g (14oz) tin of chopped tomatoes or 500g (1lb) fresh tomatoes, skinned, seeded and chopped

Sea salt to taste
Juice of 1 lemon
Fresh coriander chopped to garnish

First soak your pulses in a bowl, cover with boiling water and leave for about 3-4 hours. Alternatively you could cover in cold water and leave overnight. They are ready to cook when their drained, rehydrated weight is about double their dried weight. In this case, they should weigh about 1kg (2lb).

To cook the pulses pop them in a pressure cooker with the onion, carrot, turmeric, paprika and vegetable oil. Submerge in boiling water. Bring to pressure and cook them for 5 minutes. Allow the pressure to reduce naturally. Open up the cooker and you should have delightfully mushy pulses. If they are not, just bring them back up to pressure and cook for a little more. If they are too wet, just simmer off the water for a bit from the open pan, stirring frequently so they do not stick.

If you do not have a pressure cooker, pop the pulses, vegetables and spices in a saucepan. The vegetable oil is not needed. Cover with water and simmer until tender, stirring so they do not stick. If they look dry, stir in a little hot water. They could take anywhere between 25 and 60 minutes to cook, depending on their age. In both cases, mash the vegetables into the pulses. Put the pulse paste to one side.

In a wok or deep frying pan heat the vegetable oil over a medium-high heat. Scatter in the seeds and stir around till they pop. Add the onions and fry until they just take some colour. Add the garlic and ginger and fry for 30 seconds, then add the spices and fry for 1 minute, stirring all the time.

Pour in the tomatoes and stir well so everything is combined. Then add as much of the pulse paste as you fancy for your appetite. Stir well to mix and heat through. Sprinkle salt and lemon juice to taste and garnish with coriander.

VEGETABLE CURRY

Paste
6 shallots or 1 red onion, roughly chopped
3 garlic cloves (or quantity to taste)
20g (¾oz) knob of ginger, roughly chopped
Chillies (to taste)
A big bunch of coriander stalks, roughly chopped, save the leaves
Zest and juice of 1 lime (or lemon)

The rest
Vegetable oil
Vegetable stock
Coriander leaves (see above)
For 4 you'll need 1-1.5kg (2-3lbs) of mixed vegetables. Use more and have seconds next day.

This recipe is a doddle to put together and a great way of using your seasonal veg. Paint pictures and choose contrasting colour, texture and shape combinations of vegetables you have available. The speed with which this cooks means that we'll change round the normal method and add the curry paste to the browned veg. There are no powdered spices in this recipe.

Separate your vegetables into mushrooms, green and others. You'll brown the 'others' and pop the 'green' in later in the cooking. Cook this in a deep sauté pan or a saucepan.

You'll need a food processor or blender. Cut the paste ingredients into rough chunks just so the food processor or blender can cope with them better. Tip them into your machine and process until you have a paste.

Wash and scrub the vegetables. Peel anything that doesn't scrub up well. Cut into rough chunks, dice or batons. I wouldn't make anything much smaller than about 1.5cm (½in) dice or equivalent as they may just fall apart in cooking.

Heat 2 tablespoons of oil in your saucepan over a medium-high heat. Brown any vegetables that are not mushrooms or green vegetables in the oil. Stir occasionally to prevent too much sticking but allow them to sit so they pick up colour.

If you're using mushrooms, add these next and sauté until they just lose their firmness.

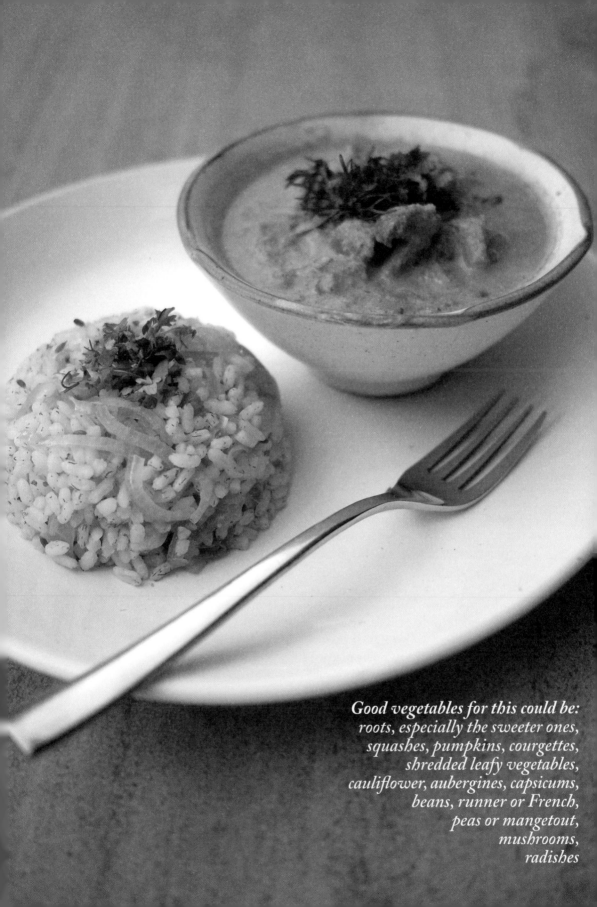

Good vegetables for this could be:
roots, especially the sweeter ones,
squashes, pumpkins, courgettes,
shredded leafy vegetables,
cauliflower, aubergines, capsicums,
beans, runner or French,
peas or mangetout,
mushrooms,
radishes

Add a good dollop of your curry paste and stir until it's fragrant and you hear a 'picking' sound.

Pour in enough stock to just cover the vegetables and bring to a simmer. Simmer until the vegetables begin to get tender, poke them with a sharp knife to see.

Once they are getting to the stage where they are nearly cooked to your satisfaction, add the green vegetables, stir well, bring back to simmer and cook until tender.

Serve garnished with the coriander leaves.

Accompaniments

I think plain white basmati is great with this. Also chunky, robust bread: a wholemeal or rye. Hot pickles or chutneys, especially home made, would also be a tangy counterpoint.

Variations and garnishes

In the curry paste you can use basil stalks or mint leaves instead of, or in addition to, the coriander stalks. Then use the leaves of one or more to garnish.

Before you pour the stock in to the pan, you could add a tin or diluted block of coconut milk. To continue the Thai theme, you could add nam pla (fish sauce) or shrimp paste at this time too.

Tofu is great with this as well. Fry in a little oil before you brown the vegetables and remove. Fold the tofu back into the curry with about 10 minutes cooking time left.

If you want to de-veggy the meal, thinly sliced chicken breast could partner with the vegetables or you could add prawns or mussels with the green veg at the end.

Onions fried until they are crisp with some cumin seeds and then scattered on to the curry at the end would make a great garnish.

FISH CURRY

Cut the fish fillets into 4 single portion sizes or large bite sized pieces. Rub some of the salt and turmeric over the fish and put to one side. You can use any left over salt/spice mix later.

Blitz the onion, garlic, ginger and coriander stalks in a processor until you have a smooth paste. You may need to use a little water to help the paste get going.

Heat 2 tablespoons of vegetable oil in a large frying or sauté pan over a medium heat. Add the fennel and mustard seeds and fry until the mustard seeds start to pop.

Add the onion, garlic, ginger paste. Be careful because it will spit. Stir fry until the liquid evaporates and the onion colours slightly.

Stir in the ground coriander and any of the salt/turmeric mix that is left and stir-fry for 1-2 minutes. Tip in the chopped tomatoes and stir well to make sure all is mixed well.

Place the fish in the pan and poach in the sauce for 10 minutes or so until the fish flakes easily.

Check seasoning and add salt if needed.

Serve garnished with the coriander leaves roughly chopped. Now how easy was that?

800g (30oz) of seasonal, sustainable white fish: fillets or steaks
Salt to taste
1tbsp ground turmeric
Vegetable oil
1 onion, roughly chopped
2 cloves garlic
20g (¾oz) ginger
1tsp fennel seeds
1tsp yellow mustard seeds
1tsp ground coriander
1 x 400g (14oz) tin of chopped tomatoes
20g (¾oz) fresh coriander, stalks and leaves roughly separated.

A great garnish for this dish is shredded basil and mint

Accompaniments

Cumin roti (see page 138) to mop up the gorgeous juices would be good. And try some chard, quickly stir fried with garlic slices, grated ginger and finely chopped fresh chilli.

FISH CURRY VEGETABLE VARIATIONS

Any of your green summer vegetables would be ideal cooked through the sauce. So try French or runner beans sliced; mangetout, sliced in thin strips length ways or into chunks cross ways or shredded lettuce. Other leafy vegetables such as chards, spinach, beetroot leaves, turnip tops work well. Try grated courgettes, kohl rabi or carrots for an interesting texture and flavour boost.

CHICKEN & LENTIL CURRY

This is one of my favourite curry recipes. It's fragrant, filling and very easy to prepare. You could make it for a midweek meal, or prepare for dinner guests with some small garnishes. I think it's best made with leg portions because the meat is more juicy. I've given generous quantities for four. You could also use wild rabbit or pheasant for a very sustainable meal.

You'll need a large saucepan to cook this in.

Fry the nigella and cumin seeds in a tablespoon of the oil until they start to pop.

Add another 1-2 tablespoons of oil to the pan and add the onion, garlic, ginger and coriander stalks. Stir-fry for 5 minutes or so over a medium-high heat until the onion is lightly coloured.

Add the cayenne or dried chilli, ground coriander and turmeric and stir-fry over a medium heat for 1-2 minutes until they are fragrant.

Tip in the lentils and coat in the oil and spice mix. If used, add the tomatoes. Give it a good stir, bring to a fast simmer and cook for 5 minutes to thicken slightly.

Add the chicken pieces and enough stock to cover everything. **Do not** add any salt at this stage because it may make the lentils tough. Bring to the boil and simmer gently for at least 40 minutes, stirring occasionally so the bottom does not catch. The chicken should be tender and the lentils dissolved.

Check the seasoning and add salt to taste. Stir through the garam masala and serve garnished with the coriander leaves.

4 chicken leg portions, skinned and, if preferred, boned and cut into bitesized pieces
Vegetable or groundnut oil
1tbsp nigella seeds (also known as kalonji)
1tsp cumin seeds
2 medium onions, finely chopped
4 cloves garlic, finely chopped or grated
20g (¾oz) ginger, finely chopped or grated
20g (¾oz) bunch coriander, leaves picked off and stalks finely chopped
Cayenne pepper or dried chilli (to taste, try first with half tsp)
1tbsp ground coriander
1tsp ground turmeric
300g (10oz) red split lentils (washed and drained)
1 x 400g (14oz) tin of chopped tomatoes or 500g (1lb) fresh tomatoes, peeled, de-seeded and roughly chopped (optional)
About 1.5 litres (6 cups) of chicken stock or water
½tsp garam masala (optional)

Accompaniments

This is great served with just plain basmati rice or roti (see page 138) and a salad. A buttery alternative could be onion pilaf.

VEGETABLE VARIATIONS

Carrots

These can be added as small dice to the onion, garlic and ginger at the beginning. Or you could add larger dice or batons when you cook the chicken. They bring sweetness and texture to the dish too.

Courgettes

These can be whatever size you fancy, diced or in rings. Added within the last 5-10 minutes of cooking time, they will retain some crunch. Use different coloured courgettes for a nice effect.

Squash or pumpkin

You can add these peeled and diced (dice will need to be 2cm / ¾in or more, otherwise they will just melt into the sauce). Stir-fry in the onion/spice mixture over a medium-high heat so they brown: this will give an even sweeter flavour.

Peas

Fresh or frozen peas are a delight in curry. Scatter into the dish in the last 5-10 minutes of cooking.

French or runner beans

Add to the curry in the last 5-10 minutes of cooking.

GREATER GARNISH

To make the meal a bit extra special you can add an extra embellishment. Start this once the chicken and lentils are simmering.

Vegetable oil
1 or 2 onions, peeled, cut in half from root to top and thinly sliced into half rings
1tsp cumin seeds
1tsp nigella seeds

Pour enough oil to cover the base of a frying pan and provide a depth of about 2mm (^{1}/$_{10}$in). Add the onions, stir and make sure the half-rounds are separated into individual strands. Cook the onion over a medium heat for 20-30 minutes, stirring occasionally, until the onions are brown all over. Take out the onions and drain them on kitchen paper.

Right before you are ready to serve, add another 2 tablespoons of oil to the pan and put on a medium-high heat. Tip in the spices and shake the pan until they pop and release their fragrance.

Tip the spiced oil onto the top of the cooked chicken and lentils and garnish with the fried onions.

LAMB & NETTLE CURRY

Vegetable or groundnut oil
1kg (2lb) lamb shoulder, boned
and cut into bite sized pieces
2 large onions, roughly
chopped
6 cloves garlic
40g (1½oz) ginger, skin scraped
and cut into big chunks
1 or 2 fresh green or red chillies,
roughly chopped (you need
to have a taste of a little bit
from the middle of a chilli to
test the heat so you can
estimate how much to use)
3 bay leaves, edges of leaves torn
1tbsp ground coriander
1tsp ground cumin
1tsp ground cinnamon
½tsp ground cardamom
Salt to taste
1kg (2lb) young nettle tops
or spinach, well washed and
coarsely chopped

Optional
1 or 2 x 400g (14oz) tins of
chopped tomatoes

or

500g-1kg (1lb-2lb) fresh
tomatoes peeled, deseeded and
roughly chopped

or

100g (4oz) natural, plain yoghurt
or crème fraîche.

Lamb has a certain sweetness to it that complements the spiciness of curry. It's also a perfect foil for other ingredients. particularly green vegetables like nettles, spinach and brassicas. This curry uses the paste method from the basic curry recipe on page 67.

I've specified lamb shoulder for this recipe because it's a bit more succulent than leg. You could use leg, shoulder or loin chops, neck or fillet. This would also be great made with cubed beef or goat (they will need longer to cook). Your butcher should be happy to bone and dice the meat for you if you're not comfortable doing it yourself.

Regardless of which meat you are using, make sure it is at room temperature before you start to cook it.

You'll need a big sauté pan or saucepan to cook this in. You can complete the dish just using one pan. I use a heavy based non-stick pan to fry the meat in as I can get it very hot without the meat sticking and without using a lot of oil.

Get your pan or non-stick frying pan very hot and add a little oil. Fry the lamb cubes on a high heat. Don't stir or faff with the meat until it's brown on one side. Then turn and sear the other sides, also without faff, until the cubes are nicely browned all over. Transfer the meat to a bowl. Fry the meat in batches without overcrowding the pan.

Blitz the onion, garlic, ginger and chillies in a food processor or blender until you have a paste. You may need to add a little water to the processor to help get things going.

Next, pour 2 tablespoons of oil into the saucepan you are using to cook the meal and heat this over a medium heat. Add the paste; be careful because it will spit in the hot oil. Fry, stirring continuously until all the water has evaporated and the paste starts to colour.

Add the bay leaves, ground spices and salt and stir-fry over a medium heat for 1-2 minutes.

Pop in your reserved lamb cubes and any juices that have collected in the bowl. Stir-fry the lamb for a couple of minutes so that it is all well coated in the fragrant paste.

If you are using the tinned or fresh tomatoes, stir them in, bring to a fast simmer and allow to thicken for 5-10 minutes.

If you are using the yoghurt or crème fraîche, add it to the sauce over a low heat stirring in a tablespoon at a time. Allow each addition to be incorporated into the sauce before adding the next so that the yoghurt does not curdle. The higher fat types are less likely to curdle.

Bring the sauce up to a simmer and cook covered for 1-1½ hours until the meat is very tender. If the meat starts to stick, just add a little water and give a stir.

Once the meat is cooked, season to taste with the salt. Then fold in the chopped nettles or spinach and stir until they have fully wilted into the sauce.

If you're cooking goat, it's likely to take 2-3 hours to be tender and cubed stewing beef will take 2-4 hours.

Accompaniments
Plain basmati rice or roti (particularly wholemeal ones, see page 138) balance the sweet meat nicely.

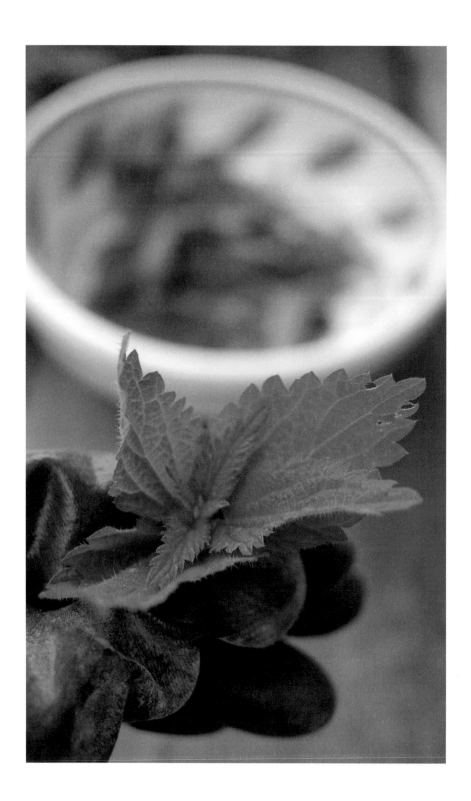

LAMB CURRY VEGETABLE VARIATIONS

Leafy vegetables
Apart from nettles and spinach, lots of other leafy vegetables will work well in this dish. Try shredded: kale, chards, cabbage, turnip tops, mustards, beetroot leaves or salad leaves that are starting to bolt.

Peas
A universal curry vegetable because of their sweetness. Add to the sauce once the lamb is cooked and simmer for 5 minutes.

Potatoes
Peel and cut the potatoes in 2-3cm (1in) cubes and add for the last hour of cooking. If you chose to use tomatoes in the sauce, it's better to par-boil the potatoes for 5 minutes and add them with 30 minutes of cooking to go. This is because the acid in the tomatoes will harden the surface of the potatoes and make it harder to cook them through.

Turnips
Turnips have an affinity with lamb. If they are small just cut into chunks and add for the last 30 minutes of cooking so they are tender. If they are larger, they may need peeling before you cut them into chunks. Cut older ones into smaller chunks so they cook more quickly. As with the potatoes, you may want to par-boil them before adding to a sauce that contains tomatoes.

GREATER GARNISHES

Almonds
Roasted flaked or whole blanched almonds. Take 50g (2oz) or so of flaked almonds, or split whole blanched almonds in half. Dry fry them in a heavy based pan, turning as necessary until they are nicely brown all over.

Yoghurt
Yoghurt is nice drizzled over the finished dish if you haven't included it as an option in the sauce.

Chopped fresh coriander or fresh mint will give a lift.

TRADITIONAL YOGHURT & MINT RAITA

150g (6oz) cucumber peeled (or use Lady's slipper achocha)
500g (1lb) natural, plain yoghurt
20g (¾oz) bunch of fresh mint or 1tbsp dried mint
Salt to taste

Optional
2 spring onions, finely chopped
½tsp cumin seeds dry roasted
¼tsp cayenne pepper

You can chop the cucumber into small dice of 5mm (¼in), slice it into thick slices, or grate it. If you have time, you can sprinkle it with a little salt and allow it to drain in a colander or sieve for 30 minutes and then rinse off the salt. This will make it crisper.

Combine all the ingredients and season to taste.

Cover and put in the fridge until you are ready to eat.

BEEF CURRY

This is a rich, slow cooked curry that is extremely easy to prepare. You could put this in a low oven or crock-pot in the morning and have a rich and fragrant curry for your evening meal.

Preheat your oven to 150°C (300°F).

This is best cooked in a lidded casserole dish that you can seal tightly to keep in moisture. You can complete the dish just using one pan. However, I tend to use a heavy based non-stick pan to brown the meat in as I can get it very hot without the meat sticking and without using too much oil.

Get your pan very hot and add a little oil. Fry the beef cubes on a high heat. Don't stir or faff with the meat until it's brown on one side. Then turn and brown the other sides, also without faff, until the cubes are nicely seared all over. Transfer the meat to a bowl. Fry the meat in small batches without overcrowding the pan.

You need to decide how much chilli to include. If you're not sure about your chillies, taste a small piece from the middle of a sample. For this recipe, I recommend you keep the chillies in larger pieces so they can be removed when you eat. If you're using fresh chillies slice them from tip to base a couple of times without cutting all the way through to expose the insides.

Heat some oil in your casserole dish over a medium-high heat. Add the onion, garlic, chillies and ginger slices. Fry and stir occasionally until the onion is lightly coloured.

Add the ground black pepper, cinnamon and salt and stir fry until fragrant.

Vegetable oil
1kg (2lb) stewing beef (shin, leg, neck, shoulder) cut into 3cm (1in) cubes
2 medium onions, finely chopped
6 cloves garlic, finely chopped
40g (1½oz) ginger, skin scraped and cut across into thin rounds
Whole fresh or dried chillies (to taste depending on heat)
1tbsp black peppercorns, dry roasted and ground in a pestle and mortar or 1tbsp freshly ground black pepper from a mill
1tbsp ground cinnamon
Salt to taste
The rind of an orange or tangerine peeled off with a vegetable peeler and with all white pith scraped off
Fresh coriander to garnish

Return the beef cubes to the pan and add the orange or tangerine zest. Pour approximately 500ml (2 cups) of water into the pan and bring to a simmer. Cover the top of the casserole with a double layer of kitchen foil and squeeze the lid on tight to trap the moisture inside.

Pop in the pre-heated oven and allow to cook for 2½-3 hours. It can easily cook for longer to suit your day. Don't peek or moisture will escape! Cook using your nose. If it smells like the casserole has run out of liquid, top it up with water.

After 2½-3 hours have a look. The beef should be meltingly tender and fragrant. There should be only a little sauce, if there's too much boil the curry for a few minutes to reduce the liquid. Remove the orange/tangerine rind, chilli pieces and ginger slices or just warn your audience they are there.

Garnish with chopped fresh coriander and serve.

VARIATIONS

You could put your potatoes or green vegetables (see overleaf) into the casserole to make this a one-pot meal. Cut the potatoes into 2-3cm (1in) chunks and give them about an hour to cook. The green vegetables can go in when the beef is cooked and can be simmered for 3 or 4 minutes on top of the stove. In both cases, you may need to add a smidge more water depending on how much liquid is in your casserole.

Accompaniments
This is just perfect with roti (see page 138) scooping up the tender meat.

As you already have the oven on Indian style baked potatoes or potato wedges are great.

A quick and easy stir-fry would enrich this dish with green seasonal veg.

Greater garnishes
The white crunch of cashew nuts provides a lovely counterpoint to the tender, dark beef. Simply roast the nuts lightly on a plate in the microwave. Give the nuts a minute at a time of power until they're a nice colour. Then remove from the plate which will be very hot and continue to brown them. Alternatively, the nuts can be dry fried, or fried with a little oil and salt in a frying pan, tossing frequently.

INDIAN STYLE
BAKED POTATOES

If you want to leave the potatoes whole, prick them with a fork all over so that any steam can escape when they cook. Or cut the potatoes in wedges.

Dry the potatoes well.

Put the oil in a small bowl and mix in the other ingredients. Use your hands or a brush to coat the potatoes with the oil. Pop the potatoes in the oven on a baking tray with the curry. Depending on their size, the whole potatoes will need about 1½ hours to cook and the wedges 35-45 minutes. Test with a slim knife. If it goes through the thickest parts easily, the potatoes are cooked. If there is any resistance, they need a bit longer.

1 large potato per person, scrubbed clean
2tbsp vegetable oil
1 or 2 cloves of garlic to taste, finely chopped or grated
1tsp turmeric
½tsp ground cumin
Salt to taste

STIR FRIED GREEN VEG

Put the oil in a pan or wok big enough to hold the vegetables on a high heat.

Throw in the mustard seeds and fry till they pop.

Put in the garlic and shredded vegetables and fry, stirring continuously until the vegetables are wilted and tender. Season and serve immediately.

500g (1lb) washed and shredded green leafy vegetable (cabbage, kale, pak choi, Chinese cabbage, mustard greens, turnip tops or cima di rapa)
2tbsp vegetable oil
1tbsp yellow or brown mustard seeds
1 or 2 garlic cloves finely chopped
Salt to taste

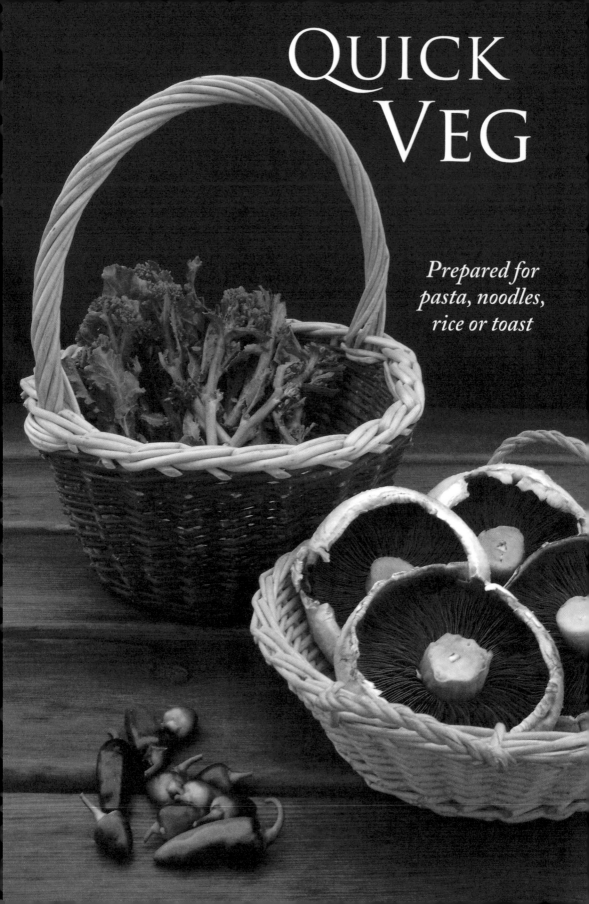

QUICK VEG

Prepared for pasta, noodles, rice or toast

In The Permaculture Kitchen you do the minimum to vegetables to create fresh, vibrant, tasty meals in about the time it takes for you to cook your pasta, rice or toast.

The quantities of the ingredients in these recipes really depend on your appetite and what you have available. So I'll give you some generalised quantities per person.

For pasta, noodles and rice, I usually work on 75-100g (3-4oz) per person. For hungrier mouths, 150g (5oz) per person is a feast.

The best pan to cook these recipes in is a sauté pan with lid. You can use a frying pan with lid or improvise using foil, greaseproof paper or a plate.

PURPLE SPROUTING BROCCOLI

A large handful of fresh purple sprouting broccoli or other brassica shoots, leave whole or cut into bitesized pieces
A garlic clove (or more), peeled and thinly sliced or finely chopped
A fresh chilli, thinly sliced or finely chopped or a pinch of dried chilli flakes
Stalks from some fresh parsley or coriander, chopped
2-6 anchovy fillets

For the western version with pasta
Extra virgin olive oil
Salt and freshly ground black pepper, to taste
Flat leaved parsley leaves to garnish, roughly chopped

For the eastern version with rice or noodles
Groundnut oil
Sesame oil
Soy sauce or oyster sauce to taste
Fresh coriander leaves, roughly chopped

This wonderful vegetable is one of the first to appear in the New Year and can crop on well into the summer. It partners perfectly with garlic, chilli, anchovies and parsley: choose which you like best. It goes well with pasta. For a more oriental feel, you can partner it with soy or oyster sauce and fresh coriander and serve with noodles.

Put your pasta to boil or rice on to cook. Soak your noodles in boiling water for 4 minutes or as directed. Drain.

Heat the oil in a sauté or frying pan over a low-medium heat. Pop in the garlic, chilli, anchovies or herb stalks you are using. Sauté these over this gentle heat until the garlic and chilli are aromatic and the garlic colours ever so slightly, about 2 minutes. The aim is to get the oils from the garlic and chilli into your sauté oil to flavour it, not to fry the stuff so it's cooked. The anchovies when heated gently just melt and provide a wonderful umami flavour.

Once you've done this, add your purple sprouting broccoli and stir around in the flavoured oil. Pop on a lid and let the purple sprouting broccoli steam for 4-6 minutes until tender with a little bite left in it.

Season according to your eastern or western preferences.

If you are cooking pasta, drain leaving some of the cooking water with it, which will help create more sauce with the vegetables. Some hard cheese grated on top is very good indeed.

If you have noodles, a little sesame seed oil stirred through is delightful.

Serve the rice into bowls.

Take your aromatic purple sprouting broccoli and stir through your pasta or noodles, or serve prettily over your rice.

PURPLE SPROUTING BROCCOLI ALTERNATIVES

Instead of the purple sprouting broccoli, you can take exactly the same approach in The Permaculture Kitchen with the following ingredients.

Winter greens
Winter greens such as kale, chard and cabbage all love this treatment.

Courgettes
Top and tail the courgettes and chop them roughly into random sized pieces. Depending on whether you want them crisp or slightly soft you can sauté them for longer. The courgettes are scrummy on toast or scooped up with roti or pitta bread. To make this even more special, stir through some ethically caught tinned tuna and some cherry tomatoes for the last 4-5 minutes of cooking to create a more substantial meal.

'MEATY' MUSHROOM & TOMATO LATE SUMMER SPECIAL

The resulting taste of this simple sauce is surprisingly complex. Mushrooms have a meaty feel and earthy taste, which is balanced by the sweetness and acidity of tomatoes. All this is complemented by the high notes of herbs.

If you are lucky, you will have foraged some lovely wild mushrooms. If not, some meaty bought wild mushrooms such as chanterelle, puffball or parasol are great. Shop-bought organic chestnut mushrooms are good too.

The tomatoes you use should be ones with skins that you are happy to eat. Some of the plum tomatoes for 'paste' or passata have thicker skins so don't use them. I've used a wide range of cherry, salad and beef tomatoes for this, which are all fine.

This is a perfect partner for spaghetti. It would do equally well served on some toasted sourdough bread with extra virgin olive oil drizzled over.

You can cook this in a sauté pan or deep frying pan.

If you're happy you have the knife skills to start to cook this now, put on your pasta to cook or get your bread ready to toast under a pre-heated grill. If not, you can wait until you've prepared the ingredients and put the tomatoes in the sauce before you start to cook the pasta or toast.

Extra virgin olive oil
A small handful of mushrooms, sliced thickly (about 3-5mm/¼in) or broken into pieces
A small handful of parsley and/or basil leaves picked and reserved and stalks chopped
½ garlic clove peeled and finely sliced
3 anchovy fillets (optional)
A big handful of tomatoes, roughly chopped. Remove any hard cores, but don't de-seed
1 lemon zested and juiced
Salt and freshly ground black pepper to taste

Heat the olive oil in your pan over a medium heat. Add the sliced mushrooms. Cook and stir occasionally until they just give out some juice.

Add the herb stalks, garlic and anchovies and cook over the medium heat for 1-2 minutes.

Add the chopped tomatoes and cook over a high heat at first, stir them well to help them break up. Once they've started to break up, turn the heat down to medium and add the lemon zest and juice. Allow the sauce to simmer fast like this to thicken slightly. Check the seasoning and add salt and pepper to taste.

When the pasta is done drain it well and stir through the sauce.

If you're having toast, dress it with a little extra virgin olive oil and arrange the sauce over the top.

Garnish both with broken up herb leaves and some more olive oil.

GRILLED ASPARAGUS & SPRING ONIONS

This dish is wonderfully fresh, takes the absolute minimum preparation and produces a stunning result. You'll get the best taste when you use top quality fresh vegetables, olive oil and cheeses.

The shape of the vegetables means that spaghetti is an ideal accompaniment. If you want to use a shorter pasta, such as penne, you can cut the vegetables into bite sized chunks after you've grilled them.

6-8 fine spears of fresh asparagus, woody bottoms broken off (save them for veg stocks)
6-8 spring onions, washed and trimmed if necessary
Extra virgin olive oil
Salt and freshly ground black pepper
A lemon
Some tarragon *and/or* flat leaf parsley *and/or* dill, leaves picked and roughly chopped
Some parmesan *or* pecorino romano or equivalent flavourful hard cheese

Start to cook your pasta in a large pan of boiling salted water before you cook the vegetables.

Place your asparagus and spring onions in a bowl or on a plate. Swish a glug of the extra virgin olive oil over them, a squeeze of lemon juice and salt and pepper to taste.

Heat a ridged griddle or heavy based frying pan to scorching. Pop the vegetables on the griddle for a minute or so until they are tender and nicely charred. Turn them so they cook all round.

Once the pasta has cooked, drain it but make sure you keep some of the cooking water to help you make a sauce.

Toss the vegetables in the pasta adding more olive oil, lemon zest and juice, salt and pepper and grated hard cheese to taste.

Garnish with the herbs.

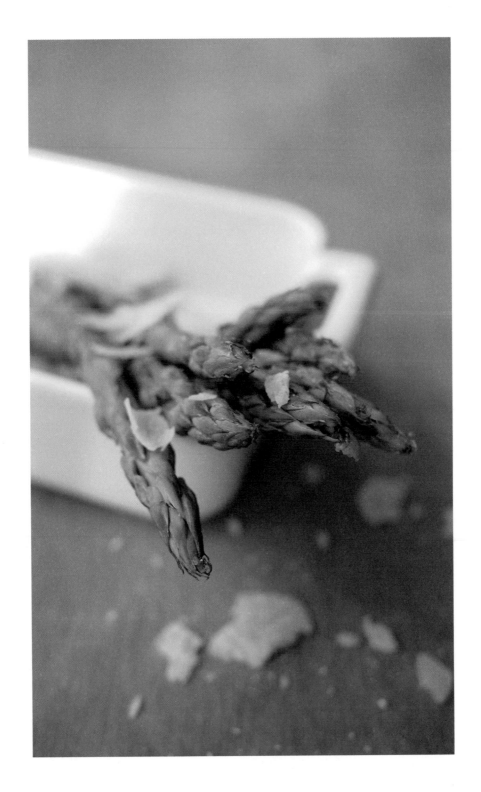

GRILLS

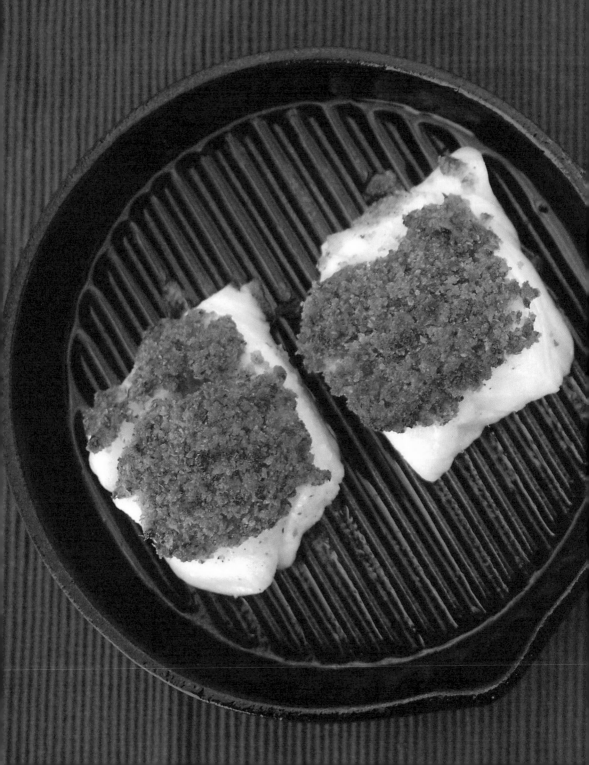

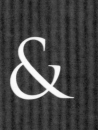

& GRIDDLES

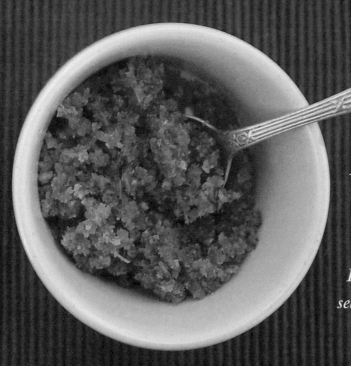

*A grill or griddled meal
can be a very quick,
healthy and succulent
way to prepare food.
It makes the best of fresh
seasonal ingredients with
minimal preparation.*

GARLIC & HERB COURGETTES

This method of cooking fresh vegetables uses a high heat to give a wonderful smoky finish to the natural sweetness of the vegetables, leaving a delightful crunchy texture. It's suitable for lots of different produce and a great way to use gluts or to combine a few different veg when you don't have many of each.

Courgettes, washed if needed, topped and tailed and cut into 3-5mm (¼in) thick slices lengthwise
Garlic cloves, peeled and left whole or crushed lightly, halved if very large
Sea salt and freshly ground black pepper to taste
Extra virgin olive oil
Vinegar, white *or* red wine, cider *or* balsamic
Thickly sliced sourdough, ciabatta or foccacia to serve *or* your favourite cooked pasta, freshly drained

If you can, use different varieties of courgette to mix colours and textures. The whole garlic is smokily sweet.

I'm not going to give detailed quantities because it really depends on your taste, appetite and the available ingredients.

This is best cooked on a stove top griddle or barbecue to get the smoky flavours. You can also sear it under a grill or in a frying pan.

Pop the sliced courgettes into a bowl. Sprinkle over the garlic and season with salt and pepper. Moisten with olive oil so that the courgettes are just coated (not drowned) and sprinkle over a little vinegar. Give it all a good mix with your hands or a spoon. Use immediately or leave for an hour for the flavours to mingle.

If you want to serve this stirred through pasta, get your pasta on the go so that it is just about ready when the vegetables are cooked.

Heat your chosen cooking method to high and turn on the extractor fan or open a window. Spread the courgettes and garlic out evenly on the hot surface. Allow to colour on one side. Give them a press to make sure you have good contact with the hot surface. Then turn over and grill the other side. This should take no longer than about 5-6 minutes.

Set to one side. Then toast your bread on the hot griddle and pile your vegetables on top. If you're using pasta, drain then stir through the vegetables and check seasoning. In either case, drizzle with some more extra virgin olive oil and tuck in.

ALTERNATIVES & VARIATIONS

Vegetables
Baby globe artichokes
French beans
Baby carrots
Cauliflower florets
Chard ribs
Chicory
Baby leeks
Mangetout peas
Parsnip thinnings
Thinly sliced sweet peppers
Radishes (halved)
Spring onions
Tomatoes, whole cherry or halved

Herb options
Pop these in the marinade and/ or garnish your meal just before you eat
Basil, torn
Coriander leaves
Dried oregano
Finely chopped fresh rosemary leaves
Parsley
Thyme leaves

Seasoning options
A pinch of dried chilli flakes, or a splash of chilli oil (optional) in with the marinade
Finely chopped anchovies
Finely chopped pancetta, lardons or smoked streaky bacon
Finely diced chorizo or other cured meats
Tinned tuna chunks

Cheeses
These are great added as a garnish before you serve and give some real punch to the dish
Finely grated parmesan, pecorino or other hard cheese
Feta cheese broken into lumps
Grilled halloumi
Blobs of soft goats cheese or fresh ricotta

GRILLED POLLACK
WITH PERSILLADE CRUMBS

In this recipe the beautiful fresh fish is contrasted with a flavourful crunch made from items in your store cupboard. It's a dish you can have on your plate in 15 minutes with a simple salad or steamed vegetables and some potatoes or noodles.

Look for chunky pollack fillets and make sure they are pin-boned. Try to leave the skin on as this provides extra flavour and holds the fillet together. Some like to eat crispy skin too.

150-200g (5-7oz) pollack fillet (or other sustainable white fish) patted dry
1tbsp persillade or pesto or similar herb paste (see page 154 for ideas)
3-4tbsp breadcrumbs
Extra virgin olive oil
Salt and freshly ground black pepper

Cook on a good baking tray, griddle or frying pan that you are happy to pop in the oven.

Turn the grill to high. In a bowl, combine the herb paste with the breadcrumbs. Loosen with a little more olive oil if it's too thick to spread.

Lightly oil the skin side of the fish and season with salt and pepper. Pile some herb-breadcrumb paste evenly on the fish fillet(s). Drizzle over a little olive oil.

Fresh fish really benefits from this quick cooking method

Heat the tray/griddle/pan on the hob until it's very hot. Place the fish skin side down. After about 5 minutes, you should start to see the flesh changing from translucent to white.

Slide under your hot grill. It needs to be about 100mm (4in) away at least or the top will burn before the fish is cooked through. Leave the fish under the grill for about 5-7 minutes until it's just cooked through and flakes easily when tested with a knife or fork. Serve immediately.

GRILLED SALMON WITH HONEY & MUSTARD DRESSING

Salmon from sustainable sources has a wonderful flavour, the dressing cuts through the oiliness and the whole grain mustard provides a nice crunch. You can finish this in the oven if it's already on for something else. If not, just cover your pan and let the steam and retained heat do the work.

Ideally use a chunky piece of fillet from the head end of the fish. If you're using tail fillets, overlap or sandwich them so they have the thickness of the head end.

This recipe will also work well for grey mullet or mackerel.

Mix together the mustard and honey. This will be easier if the honey is a bit warm. Then whisk in the orange rind and juice until well combined. Stir in the coriander leaves. Season to taste.

Slather the dressing over the top of the salmon.

Cook according to one of the method options below.

Meanwhile, mix the yoghurt or crème fraîche with the dill.

Serve garnished with a little more fresh coriander leaves and some dill sauce on the side.

4 x 200g (7oz) salmon fillets, pin boned and patted dry
1tbsp whole grain mustard
1tbsp runny honey
1 orange, rind finely grated
3tbsp juice freshly squeezed from the orange
2tbsp chopped fresh coriander leaves
Sea salt and freshly ground black pepper to taste

Garnish
More chopped coriander
150ml (10tbsp) natural yoghurt or crème fraîche or a mix
2tbsp dill tops

The fish changes colour as the heat penetrates the flesh, so you have instant feedback on how cooked things are

SALMON COOKING METHOD OPTIONS

The Permaculture Kitchen is about flexibility and minimising energy usage. So choose your method according to what you have available and what else is already being used.

Frying pan

Start off the fish in the hot pan, skin side down. Cook until the fish changes colour half way up the thickness. Then turn over and finish off. This gives you a nice crusty top to the fish.

Start off the fish in a hot pan for 2-3 minutes to get things going. Then turn down the heat and cover the pan with a lid, or some foil or greaseproof paper, a newspaper or another pan. Then steam the fish until it's cooked through and flakes easily.

Oven tray

If you have other things on to cook in the oven, you can use the heat and warm up a tray or pan in the oven. Put your fish on the hot tray/pan and pop in the oven for 10 minutes or so.

Steamer

This is a nice gentle way to cook fish. It's especially useful if you already have a pan of water for some veg on the go. Put the fish onto a small plate or bowl and pop in a steamer pan, bamboo steamer, colander or sieve. Cover this with a lid, foil or cloth and steam for 10-15 minutes or until cooked through.

Sesame style

Mix up 3tbsp soy sauce, 1tsp sesame oil, a grated clove of garlic and 1tsp of 5-spice powder for an oriental flavour. Some finely chopped spring onions and coriander leaf would be good with this too.

Mediterranean

Mix up 3tbsp extra virgin olive oil, 1tbsp lemon juice or wine vinegar, a grated clove of garlic and 1tsp dried oregano, salt and pepper. 1 or 2 finely chopped or mashed anchovies are a delicious saline addition.

Citrus

Simply lay some finely cut rounds of lemon, orange or lime over the fish and season with salt and pepper. Fresh citrus leaves are a joy to use to sandwich the fish.

Chermoula

This Moroccan sauce is a wonderful marinade which works brilliantly on fish. See the recipe for chicken overleaf.

CHICKEN CHERMOULA

This is my version of a classic Moroccan marinade that is usually used for fish. It's a really fresh and fragrant coating. The chicken is great barbecued, grilled, griddled or roasted in the oven. So it's a really ideal dish in The Permaculture Kitchen. The quantity of marinade below will make enough to easily coat 1.5kg (3lb) of chicken. You can use cubed breast fillets if you wish, I think the legs are more succulent. I make more than I need for the meal to make sure I have leftovers.

Chicken breast, thigh and drumstick (1 per person)
3 or more cloves garlic
2tbsp ground cumin
1tbsp smoked paprika
A small bunch coriander leaves or 1tbsp ground coriander
A small chilli or pinch of cayenne pepper
Zest and juice of a lemon or a preserved lemon
Olive oil
Sea salt to taste

The easiest way to make up the marinade is to put all the ingredients in a food processor and whizz them up. Use enough olive oil to make a thickish paste.

Alternatively, you can roughly chop the garlic and then smash it up with a little of the salt in a mortar and pestle or on your chopping board. Finely chop the coriander leaves, chilli and preserved lemon. In the mortar or a bowl mix the other ingredients together (apart from the olive oil) until they are thoroughly combined. Add olive oil to loosen the mixture so you have a thick paste. This mixture will keep in the fridge for a good few days.

Put your chicken portions into a bowl and coat with some or all of the marinade. Then allow to marinate for as long as you have time for – up to 12 hours or overnight.

The precise cooking times will depend on the exact nature of your heat source. See guidelines opposite. You need to make sure there is no sign of pinkness in the middle of the cooked portions. A moderate heat is better than high heat which would burn the outside before the middle is cooked.

To barbecue, griddle or grill them, cook over a moderate heat for 20-30 minutes turning often. If you want to cook them on a barbecue, make sure the coals are grey with no flames. Use a water spray bottle to douse any flames caused by the juices.

Roast them in a moderate oven at 180-200°C (350-390°F) for 30-40 minutes.

Served garnished with more chopped, fresh coriander and freshly squeezed lemon or lime juice.

Accompaniments

This is great served with salad in pitta breads or wraps, or on top of couscous or rice.

I love to make extra so that I can have it cold the next day. It is good as a poultry style burger in a bun, sandwich filling or inside a salad filled pitta bread. They are also great sliced and served dressed with warm or room temperature pasta.

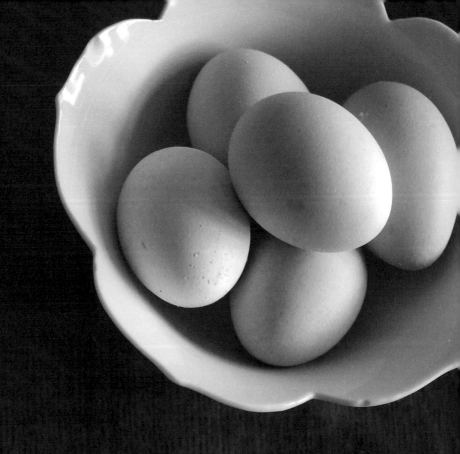

EGGS ARE
EASY

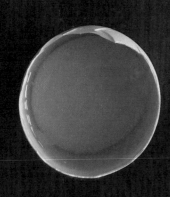

Eggs are fabulous fast food. They are nutritionally very valuable and contain protein, vitamins A, B and D, iron and calcium. Egg laying chickens are great for The Permaculture Kitchen garden too: they produce eggs, recycle vegetable waste and pests, produce great manure and are fun to be with.

If you keep chickens, it's possible that you'll experience the feast and famine of egg production. During the spring and summer the chickens lay well and it can be difficult to keep up with what they produce. Then the older chickens start to moult in the autumn and stop laying. Production restarts soon after the winter solstice.

One solution to the egg gap is to freeze some of the surplus eggs in the high time. We take 6 eggs, whisk them and keep them in freezer bags. You can add a little salt if you wish which prevents the yolks from thickening. Just defrost overnight and use as normal. They look a bit strange when they come out, but they whisk up OK and are ideal for dishes like these.

I like to use eggs with seasonal ingredients to make fast and easy meals. These meals are in the tradition of the Spanish tortilla, Italian frittata and the Middle Eastern kookoos and eggehs. My main reference for the Middle Eastern dishes is Arto der Haroutunian's *Vegetarian Dishes of the Middle East*.

These dishes are cooked with great energy efficiency because you use the best heat source available. If an oven is on for something else, the dish can be cooked there. If not, you can cook it on the hob and turn over, or start on the hob and finish under a grill.

It's worth making a big pan's worth so you can have a free 'no-cook' meal later on or have them as nibbles as these dishes are delicious cold too. They are ideal for a family main meal or to cut into slices for a party. Try topped with cheese and grilled too.

I'm giving you versions for spring/summer, autumn/winter, potato and herbs and a foraged nettle one. Hopefully, this should help you see what the principles are so that you can then make up your own versions.

SPRING & SUMMER EGGEH

About 8 medium eggs (2 per person)
A small bunch of fresh herbs, choose 1 or more from: mint, coriander, parsley, thyme, dill, chives, finely chopped (or about 1-2tsp in total of dried thyme, mint or dill)
1tsp paprika
Sea salt and freshly ground black pepper
1 onion, chopped finely
2 cloves garlic, sliced finely
Olive oil

A small handful each of
Baby carrots, or a bigger carrot cut into batons
Broad beans
Baby courgettes cut into rounds, or a larger courgette cut into batons

Make these eggehs with what you have to hand, the ingredients are just a suggestion.

If you intend to use the oven to cook this, it needs to be preheated to 180°C (350°F) with the shelf in the middle.

If the broad beans are big then blanch them in some boiling salted water for 2 minutes. Drain and refresh them in cold water and take off the outer shell.

Break the eggs into a bowl. Add the finely chopped herbs, paprika and season. Stir or whisk until all the ingredients are thoroughly combined. Set to one side.

In a pan or dish that you can use on the hob, under the grill or in the oven, put a glug of olive oil and heat over a medium heat.

Add the onions and garlic and sauté gently until the onion is tender. If you wish, add the carrots and courgettes and sauté for 2-3 minutes stirring frequently. Then add the broad beans.

Make sure that the ingredients are evenly spread in the dish and pour over the egg and herb mixture.

Pop the dish into the pre-heated oven for 30-40 minutes until the top is lightly brown and the eggeh is just firm to the touch. Then serve.

Or if you are cooking on the hob, turn the heat down to low and cover the dish with a lid, some foil, greaseproof paper or a newspaper. Cook for 15 minutes until the eggeh sounds like it's just browning underneath.

Finish off the dish by grilling for about 5-10 minutes until the top is golden and the eggeh is firm to the touch.

Otherwise, you can turn the eggeh out onto a plate, re-oil the pan and slip the eggeh back in for 10-15 minutes until it is firm to the touch. You may find it easier to cut the eggeh into portions and turn these individually back into the pan.

AUTUMN & WINTER EGGEH

Steam or boil the potatoes for roughly 10-15 minutes, until they are just tender. Drain and slide back into the pan so they can air dry while you make the rest.

Cut the ribs from the chard, finely chop and keep separate. Roughly shred the leaves and keep to one side.

Break the eggs into a bowl. Season with the salt, pepper and nutmeg to taste.

Heat a good glug of olive oil in your pan or dish over a medium heat. If you are using bacon, fry this gently in the oil until the fat renders and the bacon starts to colour.

Add the leek/onion, garlic, vegetable ribs and chilli to the oil, sauté gently until the vegetables are tender. Stir in the mushrooms and fry over a medium heat until they just start to soften.

Pour in the cider vinegar. Continuously stir and scrape the bottom of the pan until the vinegar is almost evaporated.

Then cook as you would the spring/summer version.

3 medium potatoes, scrubbed or peeled and cut into 2-3cm (1in) chunks
100g (4oz) smoked streaky bacon or similar, finely sliced (optional)
A small handful of: chard, spinach, kale, beetroot leaves or foraged greens; or a mixture, washed and well drained and dried
Halved green or red cherry tomatoes, or tomato chunks
Chestnut mushrooms or foraged mushrooms
Fresh herbs, one or a mixture, leaves picked and roughly chopped and any soft stems retained and finely chopped
Olive oil
1 leek or onion, coarsely chopped
3 cloves garlic finely sliced
1 fresh chilli (or to taste) finely sliced or finely chopped
2-3tbsp apple cider vinegar
About 8 medium eggs (2 per person)
Sea salt and freshly ground black pepper to taste
½ nutmeg finely grated

SEPHARDIC OMELETTE WITH NETTLES

25g (1oz) unsalted butter
Small onion, finely chopped
2-3 garlic cloves, crushed and
finely chopped
125g (4oz) mushrooms cleaned
and sliced, or (best) 50g (2oz)
dried porcini mushrooms
soaked in warm water and
squeezed dry
4 free range eggs
60ml (4tbsp) milk
150g (5oz) young nettle tops,
washed, dried and
chopped coarsely
150g (5oz) grated or crumbled
cheese (feta is nice or use a
cheese of your choice)
Fresh parsley and chives,
small handful of each,
finely chopped
Salt and freshly ground
pepper to taste

This recipe illustrates just how easy and tasty it is to use foraged vegetables in your diet. You can use other foraged greens, spinach or kale instead of nettles.

Pre-heat your oven to 190°C (370°F). You'll need a lightly buttered casserole dish about 25cm (10in) in diameter or similar.

Melt the butter in a deep frying pan or wok.

Sauté the onion and garlic on a medium heat until the onion takes on some colour around the edges.

Add the mushrooms. You may need to use slightly more butter or some olive oil with fresh mushrooms. Sauté until just tender but before they give up juice.

Add the nettles, stir frequently and allow them to wilt.

Put to one side and allow the vegetable mix to cool a little.

In a bowl crack in the eggs and milk and beat gently. Mix in the remaining ingredients and the onion/mushroom/nettle mixture. Pour into your casserole dish.

Bake in the oven for 30-40 minutes until golden on top.

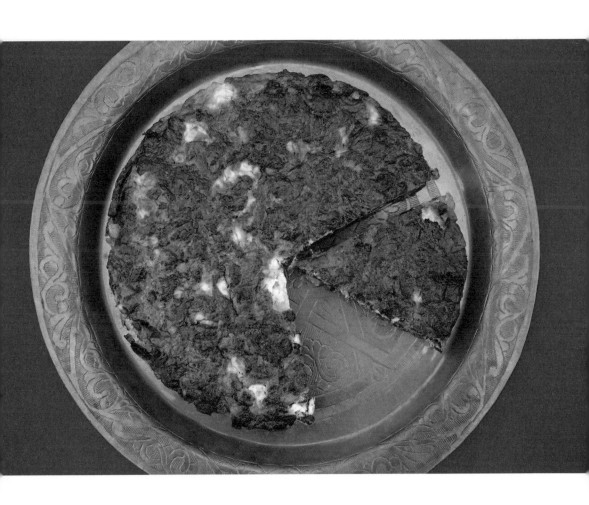

POTATO EGGEH

2 large floury potatoes, peeled boiled and mashed without butter or milk
Olive oil
1 small onion, a medium leek or a small bunch of spring onions, finely chopped
1 or 2 cloves garlic, finely chopped
A small bunch of parsley or coriander, leaves picked and chopped, stems finely chopped
6 eggs
1tsp dried dill
1tsp smoked paprika
Sea salt and freshly ground black pepper to taste

This is a delightfully tasty and surprisingly light eggeh. It's great with a salad and some yoghurt raita.

This one is best cooked in the oven. Preheat it to 180°C (350°F). Butter an oven dish well.

Give the pan you used to cook the mashed potatoes a bit of a rinse and dry. Heat the olive oil in the pan over a medium heat. Add the onion, leek, spring onions, garlic and herb stalks. Sauté gently until tender. Then allow them to cool a little before you add them to the eggs in the next step or you'll start to cook the eggs before you mean to.

Meanwhile, break the eggs into a bowl and beat them well. Add the mashed potato, herb leaves, dried dill, paprika and season to taste. Beat until the mixture is thoroughly combined.

Once the onions etc. have cooled a little stir them into the egg mixture.

Pour into the prepared oven dish and bake for 40-45 minutes until the eggeh is lightly browned and firm to the touch.

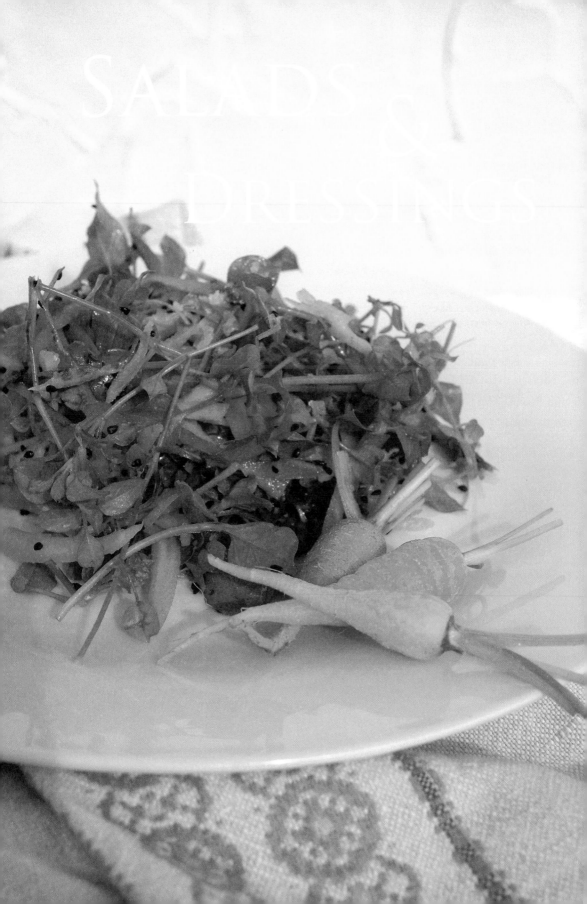

Salads are a great way to experience the seasonal joy of The Permaculture Kitchen. You can paint with the food using complementary or contrasting colours, textures and flavours. You can also eat raw, part-cooked or fully cooked salads.

You will notice the change in the weather and seasons if you prepare salads throughout the year and become more aware of what's available. You'll taste and feel the difference between young produce and those reaching maturity.

If it's an accompaniment, you need to balance it with what you plan to serve. For example, if you plan to serve an oily fish dish, a salad with few ingredients will cut through the oil of the fish – say slivers of radish and fennel in a simple lemon vinaigrette. With juicy grilled meat, try some buttery, soft leaves to mop up the juices.

If it's the main bit of the meal, then it may be best to go for more variety in colour, texture and tastes to appeal to the eye and taste buds alike.

You also need to decide on how to prepare the ingredients. You have three main choices for each ingredient: raw; boiled or blanched; and grilled or roasted.

Finally, before you paint with your ingredients you need to decide whether and how to dress the salad. Do you want it in the barest, skimpy clothes so its natural self can take the stage? Or do you want to clothe it in something thicker to enhance its underlying beauty? I've given a few dressing recipes at the end of this chapter.

Apart from cultivated and market bought salad ingredients, there are many ingredients you can forage for free. These seasonal contributions are really tasty and nutritious. Look out for: chickweed, nettles, bittercress, dandelion, edible flowers and more.

For your dressings to be able to stick to your ingredients, the ingredients need to be well dried as oils and water do not mix. If you don't have a spinner and want to improvise, pop the ingredients in a tea towel, pull the corners of the towel up to make a little pouch and swing it back and forward sharply. Obviously, it's best to do this outside or into the bath...

BLANCHED BEAN
& NUT SALAD

This is a great way of using a mixed harvest of beans from your garden, allotment or veg box. If you're buying in a shop or market, choose different coloured beans for an attractive platter.

Blanch the beans for just enough time to warm them through and take off any toughness. Very young fine beans of 2mm (less than ⅛in) diameter will only need a minute. Mature beans, 5mm (¼in) or over in diameter, may need 5 minutes or longer. The best thing to do is to sample the beans at intervals so that you get an idea of how long you need to cook them for.

Dress the beans while they are still warm so they really absorb the dressing.

Choose nuts you like. I think whole almonds go well, as do hazelnuts. You're after a good flavourful crunch to contrast and complement the beans.

The quantities are deliberately vague. Experiment with what you have to hand and see what you enjoy.

Two or three handfuls of (preferably mixed) French beans
A handful of whole blanched almonds or hazelnuts (or a mix)
Extra virgin olive oil
Juice of 1 lemon (and the finely grated zest too if you like)
Sea salt and freshly ground black pepper

Tail the beans. I usually don't top them unless they need it. I just rub off the flower if it's still attached. I think the fine 'comma' of the bean top looks elegant.

Roast the nuts in a heavy based pan shaking or stirring to brown them all over. You can crush or lightly chop the nuts if you'd like them a bit smaller but don't loose the lovely crunch.

Pop the beans into a pan of boiling salted water and cook to your desired degree.

Dress the beans with a good glug of olive oil, a generous squeeze of lemon juice and salt and pepper. Toss well and sprinkle with nuts and serve.

VARIATIONS

Herbs
Garnish with finely chopped parsley, tarragon or summer savory leaves.

Seeds
Use toasted sesame or sunflower seeds instead of nuts.

WARM LETTUCE, POTATO & BACON SALAD

This is comfort food par excellence. What's even better is that it's ready in a trice.

It's ultimately satisfying with some good crusty bread and a nice glass of wine. If you have super fresh eggs from local hens, then a poached egg served on top is heavenly.

You can use a whole head of one type of lettuce, or use a mixture of leaves depending on what you have available. It's a great way of using up a glut of salad leaves, especially ones that are more mature.

Your choice of potatoes will depend on what's available. You could choose waxy potatoes that hold their shape or floury potatoes that will break up a little.

A poached egg served on top of the salad is heavenly

225g (8oz) bacon, lardons or pancetta cut into rough dice or fine strips
3 cloves of garlic, peeled and finely sliced
1 head of lettuce or endive, or a mixture of leaves of about 500g (1lb) in weight
500g (1lb) potatoes scrubbed or peeled and cut into 2-3cm (1in) chunks
60ml (4tbsp) olive oil or lard or a mixture of the two
30ml (2tbsp) red wine or cider vinegar
Sea salt and freshly ground black pepper
Fresh eggs, poached (optional to serve)

Wash the salad leaves and dry well using a salad spinner and/or a tea towel. Keep the leaves to one side.

Cook the potatoes in plenty of boiling water until they are tender, about 10-20 minutes depending on size and type of potato.

Drain the potatoes in a colander and put the reserved salad leaves in the pan. Put the potatoes on top of the leaves and season with salt and pepper. Cover the pan and leave in a warm place while you make the poached eggs and the dressing.

Use very fresh eggs, less than a week old. Heat some water to a slow simmer in a pan.

WARM LETTUCE, POTATO & BACON SALAD
continued

Break the eggs into the pan. With very fresh eggs you will notice the white stays coherent around the yolk. Simmer gently for 3 minutes and take them out with a slotted spoon.

While the eggs cook make the dressing. Heat the olive oil/lard over a medium hot heat in a frying pan. Fry the bacon until the fat starts to render, then add the garlic until the bacon crisps up.

Tip the vinegar into the bacon pan. It will spit and bubble. Give a quick scrape of the bottom of the pan to loosen any residue and then quickly tip the contents of the frying pan into the leaves and potatoes.

Toss all the ingredients together well, check and adjust the seasoning.

Serve in bowl with the lightly poached egg balanced on top.

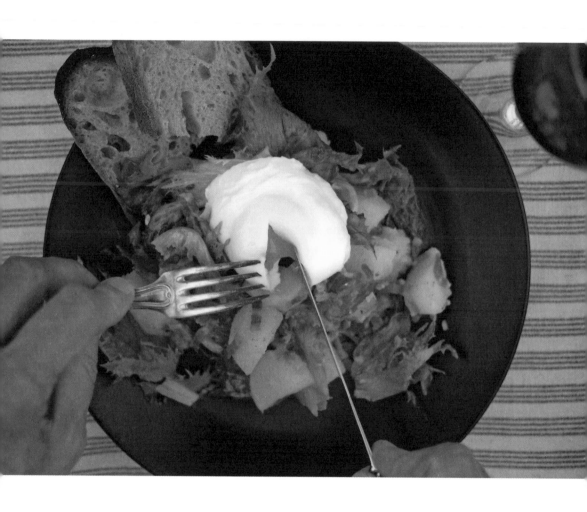

BROAD BEAN, COURGETTE, FETA & MINT SALAD

The late spring-early summer is often the time to look for something different to do with the vegetable harvest. This recipe combines seasonal produce with natural partners to create a Middle Eastern style salad. This is ideal as a side dish or eaten for a lighter meal with pitta or flat breads.

Try to use different coloured courgettes. The courgette flowers are a pretty garnish. If you don't have them, calendula, nasturtium or rose petals instead are beautiful too.

250g (8oz) broad beans shelled
100g (4oz) courgettes
5-10 courgette flower petals (or a small quantity of other edible flowers)
75g (3oz) feta cheese or similar
½ lemon, juiced
1-2tbsp extra virgin olive oil
Freshly ground black pepper
Small bunch of mint, dill or summer savory or a mixture, finely chopped

Add edible flowers like nasturtiums to salads for an extra burst of colour

Blanch the broad beans for 1-3 minutes depending on their size. If they are very small there is no need to skin them. If they are larger, take off the tough outer skin.

Top and tail the courgettes and cut into 1cm (½in) rounds.

Tear the courgette flower petals into attractive strips.

Cut the cheese into small dice of about 5mm (¼in).

Assemble all the ingredients in a bowl.

Whisk together the lemon juice, olive oil and pepper. Taste test and add more juice, oil or pepper if needed. I don't think you need any salt because of the saltiness of the feta.

Sprinkle over the finely chopped herbs and serve.

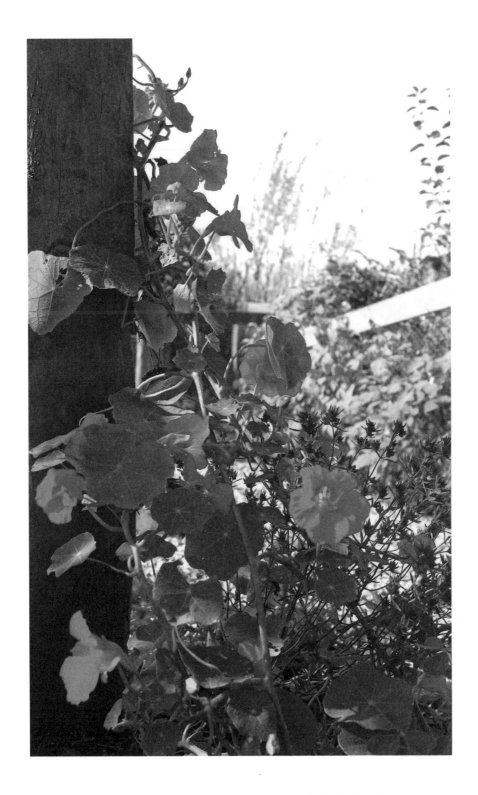

LE CRUNCH SUMMER SALAD WITH ARTICHOKES

15 medium artichokes
6 medium sized waxy potatoes
such as Charlotte, scrubbed
and cut into even sized chunks
of about 3cm (⅛in)
12 radishes, cut into even sized
chunks about 1cm (½in)
4 baby courgettes cut into 1cm
(½in) chunks
Courgette flower petals, torn
Small bunch of mixed chives,
mint and tarragon,
roughly chopped

For the dressing
45ml (3tbsp) tarragon or white
wine vinegar
135ml (9tbsp) extra virgin
olive oil
2-3 garlic cloves, peeled and
finely grated or chopped
25g (1oz) anchovies (leave out
or substitute some kalamata
or black olives for a
vegetarian version)
1tbsp Dijon mustard
Small bunch tarragon,
leaves picked
Sea salt and freshly ground
black pepper to taste

I love artichokes but it can be a real faff to prepare them. So I have worked out a very simple way to get tender hearts, faff-free.

Here they are coated in a creamy, fragrant dressing. Depending on what's available, you can paint a picture on the plate with different varieties of courgette and radish.

The dressing quantity will be more than you need. Store the remainder in a jar in the fridge, it'll keep for ages.

Boil the potatoes until tender and start to cook the artichokes (*as opposite*).

Make the dressing. The easiest way is to whizz it up in a small blender. Alternatively, chop the anchovies and tarragon very finely and then bash up with some salt and pepper in a pestle and mortar. Add the other ingredients and mix well. Taste the dressing and adjust the seasoning if necessary. Pour the dressing into a jar with a firm fitting lid.

Coat the drained potatoes with a little dressing so that they absorb some of it. When the artichokes are ready, put the rest of the vegetables into the serving bowl and mix with some more dressing so that they are generously coated but not drowned.

Garnish with the torn courgette flower petals and serve.

HOW TO PREPARE
ARTICHOKES SIMPLY

Trim the artichoke stalks so that they fit in a big saucepan.
Cover in well-salted boiling water and use a small plate
or bowl to weight the artichokes under the water.
Cover and simmer for 10-20 minutes until the biggest
artichoke is tender when you pierce its base with a
sharp knife.

Drain the artichokes and return to the pan. Cover in
cold water to cool them down.

When cool enough to handle, strip off the outer leaves.
Now they are cooked this will be really easy. Remove the
hairy bit in the middle (the 'choke') leaving you with a
beautifully tender artichoke heart. Slice or quarter the
hearts. Drop the prepared artichokes into some water
with a little lemon juice or vinegar in to stop them
going brown.

CROCSLAW

The word 'slaw' comes from the Dutch *sla* and French *salade*. It's more familiar to many of us as 'Cole-slaw' – the cole from the Latin *caulis* meaning stem, stalk or cabbage.

In The Permaculture Kitchen, grated roots and cabbages are a great way of getting the real flavour and crunch of raw vegetables. You can follow the seasons with the colours of your slaw.

A mandolin or a decent box grater are real assets for preparing slaws as they give really fine shreds. Powered food processors are quick but apart from the energy use issue, I find their results can be more inconsistent depending on how the vegetable is presented to the cutting blade.

This slaw is a summer slaw using cabbage, radish, onion and carrot: hence the name 'croc-slaw'.

200-300g (7-10oz) cabbage; use what you have to hand: a mixture of white/red/green is excellent
200g (7oz) carrots, scrubbed and topped and tailed
1 red onion peeled and halved
A handful of radishes, washed
Flat leaved parsley

Optional
Large handful of sunflower or pumpkin seeds or chopped hazelnuts

---

Shred the cabbages finely, grate the carrots coarsely and slice the red onion as finely as you can. Slice the radishes into whatever size/shape appeals to you. Pick the leaves from the parsley. Chop the stalk very finely and the leaves roughly.

Roast the seeds and/or nuts in a dry pan, stirring often until they are lightly browned.

Combine all the ingredients in a big bowl.

Dress with a thinned mayonnaise (see page 132) or thick vinaigrette (see page 129).

HOT DRESSED CHICKWEED, CARROT & KALONJI SALAD

This salad is simplicity itself. The deep green of the chickweed contrasts with the vibrant orange of the carrots and deep black kalonji seeds.

Kalonji is the Hindu/Urdu word for the seeds of the plant *Nigella sativa*. It's not the nigella plant many people have in their gardens and it's not onion seed either. You'll find it in shops with a good spice range or you can buy it as I do online.

Mix the chickweed and grated carrot in a salad bowl.

Heat the vegetable oil in a frying pan until just smoking. Scatter in the kalonji seeds and mix through the oil until they pop. This will happen very quickly so make sure you don't overcook or burn them. Tip the seeds and hot oil over the salad, pour over the orange juice and season to taste with salt. Toss the salad and tuck in.

50g (2oz) chickweed, washed and roughly chopped (or use watercress/land cress/bittercress)
2-3 medium carrots, scrubbed, topped and tailed and coarsely grated
3tbsp vegetable oil
1-2tbsp kalonji seeds
½ orange, juiced
Sea salt to taste

SEASONAL BREAD SALADS

If you make or use much real bread, you'll often have bits left over which would be a shame to waste. But in The Permaculture Kitchen, you can make them into breadcrumbs or croutons which you can freeze or keep dried. Bread can also act as the foil for some big flavours in seasonal salads.

These salads are a great way to use small harvests or leftover vegetables. In Italy this type of salad is called a panzanella.

The bread needs to be a few days old and dry. Traditionally, the bread is soaked in water or vinegar to soften it. I think that you only need to do this if it is very dry and, if so, my preference is to soak it in a little good quality red wine vinegar or sherry vinegar. Otherwise, the vegetable juices and the salad dressing should be enough to moisten the bread.

I've given you a summer and a winter recipe to illustrate the possibilities. In the winter salad, I show you how the bread is made into croutons for a deliberate crunch. This really is a very flexible and versatile dish, so feel free to play with flavours, colours and textures with your seasonal produce. For each recipe I've identified some base ingredients and some optional extras. Really anything goes, the only limit is the available produce and your imagination.

SUMMER BREAD SALAD BASE

300-400g (10-14oz) old bread roughly broken into
bitesized pieces
Red wine or sherry vinegar
500g-1kg (1-2lb) ripe tomatoes, preferably mixed
colours and shapes
1 red onion, peeled and cut in half from root to top
A big bunch of basil

DRESSING

More red wine or sherry vinegar
Extra virgin olive oil
1 or more garlic cloves, peeled and crushed with a little salt
or finely grated

INGREDIENT SUGGESTIONS

Salad leaves, cultivated or foraged
Grilled peppers, cut into strips
Blanched broad or French beans
Capers, roughly chopped
Anchovies, whole or chopped
Grilled tuna or salmon, broken into pieces or flakes
Grilled or fried bacon, pancetta, chorizo
Celery hearts, finely sliced
Artichokes, boiled and sliced or grilled
Radishes, chopped or sliced
Cheeses, parmesan, mozzarella, goat's cheese,
grilled halloumi or vegetarian alternatives
Fruit such as strawberries, peaches, nectarines

If you wish to, moisten the bread cubes in about 50ml (3tbsp) of the vinegar, water or a mixture of the two in the bowl you are using to serve the salad. You can then prepare the rest of the ingredients.

Chop the tomatoes and add them to the bread.

Slice the red onion into very fine half rings. A mandolin is perfect for this, or you can use a sharp knife or the fine blade of a food processor. It's important that the slices are fine or the taste will be too strong. Add these to the bread and tomatoes.

From here the bread, tomatoes and onions can rest while you prepare everything else.

Blanch any vegetables you have that need to be tenderised and refresh in cold water. Drain, pat dry and cut into bite sized pieces.

Slice, chop or tear the other vegetables attractively.

Mix the prepared vegetables and garlic with the salad.

Tear the basil and drape over the salad. Season with salt and pepper and dress with some extra virgin olive oil. Toss gently with your hands. Taste check the seasoning, add more vinegar, oil or salt and pepper if you need. Serve and enjoy your feast.

WINTER BREAD SALAD BASE

500g (1lb) old bread roughly broken into bitesized pieces
6 or more cloves garlic, peeled and left whole
500g (1lb) or so butternut squash or other winter squash
or pumpkin
1 or more red onion, peeled
A small bunch of mixed fresh herbs, such as
thyme, flat leaf parsley

INGREDIENT SUGGESTIONS

Chilli flakes, crushed coriander seeds, fennel seeds
or cumin seeds, for roasting vegetables
Winter salad leaves, for example radicchio, endive,
chickweed, bittercress, winter lettuce leaves
Winter greens, shredded finely
Cavolo nero
Brussels sprouts
Roots, shredded, grated or roasted chunks
Beets
Carrots
Turnips
Fresh seasonal fruit such as apples, cut into bitesized pieces
Preserved summer harvest, rehydrated where needed,
e.g. dried tomatoes and dried fruits
Peppers
Artichokes
Blanched broad or French beans
Capers, or nasturtium capers roughly chopped
Anchovies, whole or chopped
Grilled tuna or salmon, broken into pieces or flakes
Grilled or fried bacon, pancetta, chorizo
Celery hearts finely sliced
Cheeses, parmesan, mozzarella, goat's cheese, grilled halloumi
or vegetarian alternatives

SEASONAL BREAD SALADS *continued*

Pre-heat your oven to 180-200°C (350-390°F).

Slip the bread chunks into a bowl and drizzle over some of your olive oil, season with a little salt and pepper. If you want to use it, finely grate over some parmesan or other hard cheese and mix well.

Pop the bread cubes in the oven for 20 minutes or so until they are brown and crispy. Turn them over half way if you fancy. When they are finished, put them to one side and leave the oven on.

While you make the croutons, scrub and peel your squash and any root vegetables as necessary and cut them into bite-sized chunks. The red onion(s) are good roasted too, so slice them into narrow wedges and add. Leave the garlic clove(s) whole. Glug a little olive oil and vinegar over, sprinkle whatever seasonings you choose and include the spices and some of the fresh herbs. If you want to use bacon etc. then you can include this as small dice mixed in with the vegetables.

Place in the oven for 20-40 minutes until the vegetables are just tender to the point of a knife. If you are using tougher root vegetables (such as older beets or turnips) then they may benefit from par-boiling whole for up to 10 minutes so that all the vegetables roast in the same time.

Blanch any vegetables that need cooking and refresh in cold water. Drain and pat dry and cut into bitesized pieces.

Slice, chop or tear the other vegetables attractively.

Combine the croutons and vegetables with the remaining fresh herbs. Season with salt and pepper and dress with some extra virgin olive oil. You can use a basic vinaigrette for the dressing but remove the garlic if you prefer.

Toss gently with your hands. Taste check the seasoning adding more vinegar, oil or salt and pepper if you need. Serve and enjoy your feast.

BASIC VINAIGRETTE

The word comes from the French for sour-wine, *vin-aigre*. The vinegar flavours the leaves and combines with oil to help it stick to the salad.

My own preference is to start with a ratio of 1 to 3 vinegar to oil and then adjust ingredients as necessary.

Other seasonings and flavourings can also be included such as:

Keep a jar in the fridge so you'll always have some to hand

- Fresh or dried herbs
- Garlic
- Anchovies
- Mustard

You can choose vinegar or citrus juice to match the ingredients in the salad or the ingredients in its accompanying dish. I love to use tarragon infused white wine vinegar (see page 156) in dressings that go with fish and chicken salads.

I like to use a bigger flavoured extra virgin olive oil for my day-to-day vinaigrette but some people prefer neutral flavoured oil such as sunflower or a mild olive oil.

2tbsp vinegar
6tbsp vegetable or olive oil
1 clove garlic, finely grated or crushed and mashed to a paste with some of the salt
1tsp Dijon (or other) mustard
Sea salt and black pepper to taste

Combine all the ingredients in a screw top jar. Screw the lid on tight and shake vigorously until the dressing emulsifies. Keep in the fridge.

To make an elegant tarragon vinaigrette, use a tarragon infused white wine vinegar.

QUICK & SIMPLE DRESSING

½ lemon
Extra virgin olive oil – a bottle
with a spout is handy
Sea salt and freshly ground
black pepper

The very freshest leaves, full of flavour from the garden or market, don't need a complex dressing. In which case, you can just dress them quickly and simply.

The only rule with this is to put the lemon juice on first. If you put the oil on first, then the citrus juice will not stick to the ingredients and will end up in the bottom of the salad bowl.

Squeeze the lemon over the salad, catching any pips. Lightly toss, drizzle over a glug of olive oil and season to taste with the salt and pepper. Lightly toss the salad again. Taste and add anything you think you need more of. Dress the salad, don't drown it.

HONEY, MUSTARD & ORANGE DRESSING

2tbsp honey
3tbsp freshly squeezed
orange juice
1tbsp of wholegrain mustard
150ml (10tbsp) olive oil or
vegetable oil
Sea salt to taste
Finely chopped tarragon leaves
(give a bright anise taste if
available, but optional)

This dressing is good with all sorts of salads: leaves and vegetables. Salads dressed with it make a good accompaniment to grilled fish, aubergines and squashes.

Put the honey into a glass jar and stand it in some hot water. This will make it runnier and easier to mix with the other ingredients.

Pour in the orange juice and mustard and stir well or put a lid on the jar and give it a good shake. Then add the oil, salt and pepper and whisk or shake to combine and emulsify. If using, add the tarragon leaves and give another mix through.

ASIAN STYLE YOGHURT

This dressing is great on slaws instead of mayonnaise. It has bags of flavour and coats well. In its undiluted form, it's also a great marinade for chicken, fish and pork. You can stir it into soups and dhals for a creamier texture.

Whisk all the ingredients together. Start with the minimum amounts and taste as you go to get it just right.

If your dressing is too thick, thin it with some bland vegetable oil or water and give it a good whisk to blend it.

125ml (½ cup) yoghurt (low fat will give a thinner result than Greek full fat, choose what you prefer)
1 lemon or lime, zested and juiced
1-2tbsp soy sauce to taste
1 (or more) garlic cloves, finely grated/chopped or crushed to a paste
10-15g (½oz) fresh ginger, finely grated/chopped
1-2tbsp finely chopped fresh coriander

THICK GARLIC, ROSEMARY & ANCHOVY DRESSING

This is one of my favourite dressings. It's most useful when you have a salad with really bold ingredients like tuna or roast beef for example.

It's full of punchy, big flavours and makes an ideal partner for summer salads with barbecues or winter salads when you want to bring the taste of summer back again.

It's quickest made in a small food processor. You can also make it using a mortar and pestle or chop the ingredients very finely with a knife.

Put the anchovies, garlic, rosemary and lemon juice or vinegar in a food processor and whizz to a fine paste. Pour in the olive oil and whizz again to an emulsion and season to taste.

20g (1oz) anchovies in oil, drained
2 cloves garlic, peeled and roughly chopped (you can use more if you like)
2 or 3 sprigs rosemary, leaves picked and roughly chopped (my sprigs are about 10cm long)
2tbsp lemon juice or vinegar (red or white wine, or cider)
6tbsp punchy olive oil
Sea salt and freshly ground black pepper to taste

MAYONNAISE & VARIATIONS

There's a bit of mystery behind how to make mayonnaise. Here I show you two ways which really are a doddle as long as you follow these simple rules.

Homemade mayonnaise has a wonderfully rich taste, which commercial varieties cannot match. It's great as a simple dressing for potatoes or artichokes as well as a dip for raw vegetables or French fries. You can also use it as the basis for other dressings, dips or swirls with added ingredients such as chilli, paprika, breadcrumbs, fresh herbs, capers or prawns.

For people who keep chickens, mayonnaise is a delicious way of using fresh eggs. In fact, fresher eggs mean better mayonnaise as they contain more of the natural stabiliser lecithin.

Your major choice with mayonnaise is which oil to use. Your choice will affect the finished taste of the mayonnaise and its expense. I use a mix of extra virgin olive oil and neutral sunflower or olive oil. This gives a rounded flavour while keeping the cost down.

Your ingredients are best at a cool to moderate room temperature. If you've been baking all day and the kitchen feels like an oven, you will find the mayonnaise harder to make. What you are making is an emulsion of oil in water. The egg yolks and (if used) garlic and mustard help stabilise the emulsion.

There are two main methods for making mayonnaise: by hand with a whisk or pestle; or by machine with a stick blender or food processor. You use just egg yolks with the by hand method. In the machine version, you use whole eggs and the white of the eggs help to act as a buffer against the high speeds of the blades which could cause the mayo to split.

MAYONNAISE BY HAND

Whisk the egg yolk(s) and salt together until they thicken a little.

Stir in the pepper and mustard and beat with the pestle or whisk until the eggs change colour. You are making the first emulsion of the egg yolk fats with the water in the yolk and other ingredients. It's important to get this started before adding the oil.

Carefully drip the oil in at first. Beat or whisk vigorously so that it combines and disappears before you add more. Make sure you get to the sides and bottom of the bowl. You will see the colour change as you mix.

You may find it easier to rest the bowl or mortar on a damp tea towel to help keep it still.

After you've added about 75ml (5tbsp) of oil you can trickle in more but ensure you keep beating the mix well to combine the oil.

Once all the oil is added, pour in the vinegar to taste and check your seasoning. If you want to thin the mayonnaise add some more vinegar, lemon juice or some warm water. You can thicken it if you add more oil, although there is an upper limit of how much oil the eggs can hold.

If your mayo splits while you are making it, just beat a new egg yolk with a little mustard and vinegar. Very slowly beat in the curdled mayo little bit by little bit and you should be ok.

1 large or 2 small egg yolks
A large pinch of sea salt
White or freshly ground black pepper (use white if you don't want flecks in the finished mayo)
1tsp Dijon mustard
About 300ml (1¼ cups) oil (I use 50/50 olive oil and extra virgin olive oil)
1tsp white wine vinegar, or to taste (flavoured vinegars can be nice here) or you can use lemon juice

ZESTY FLAVOURS

Try 2tbsp of finely chopped coriander leaves and the zest and juice of 2 limes mixed into the mayo.

MACHINE MAYONNAISE

1 medium egg
A large pinch of sea salt
White or freshly ground black
pepper (use white if you don't
want flecks in the finished mayo)
1tsp Dijon mustard
About 300ml (1¼ cups) oil
(I use 50/50 olive oil and
extra virgin olive oil)
1tsp white wine vinegar, or to
taste (flavoured vinegars can be
nice here) or use lemon juice

This makes a slightly thinner mayonnaise.

Method: using a stick blender

Put all the ingredients in a blender goblet, jug or the bowl of your food processor.

Allow the egg to settle to the bottom. Put your stick blender to the bottom of the container and turn on. After a while, you will see the egg and some of the oil emulsify and turn white. Make sure that this is complete before gradually lifting the blender up and down through the mix to incorporate the rest of the oil. This will take about a minute in total. Check your seasoning.

Method: using a food processor

Add all the ingredients except the oil to the processor bowl. Process for a few seconds until the eggs are emulsified and change colour. Add the oil in a continuous thin stream until it's fully incorporated. Check your seasoning.

GREEN MAYO

Use a small bunch of finely chopped or puréed watercress, or cooked and puréed spinach or foraged greens such as nettles or chickweed.

TARTAR SAUCE

200ml (¾ cup) mayonnaise
3tbsp each of chopped capers,
gherkins and parsley
1 shallot, finely chopped or
small bunch chives,
finely chopped
Lemon juice to taste

This is the classic fish accompaniment.

Mix all the ingredients together and chill.

AÏOLI

Aïoli is a garlic flavoured mayonnaise sauce.

For a simple version, add 1 or more garlic cloves (to taste) mashed with the salt at the beginning of the hand method or with the eggs in the blender method.

Alternatively you can make up the mayonnaise and stir mashed garlic through.

You can achieve a less punchy and more rounded taste by using roasted garlic. Pop the whole garlic cloves in a hot oven for about 30 minutes, squeeze out the pulp and mix through. Or you can confit some peeled cloves in olive oil that is just below a simmer for 20 minutes and mash and stir this through.

Serve the aïoli with grills or barbecues, cold poached fish, salt cod dishes, eggs and raw vegetable crudités.

FRESH HERB MAYONNAISE

Once you've made the mayo, you can mix finely chopped, soft leaved herbs through the mayo to modify the flavours. 2-3tbsp are satisfactory with the basic quantity, but test for taste and texture. Try these individually or in combination:

- Basil
- Chervil
- Chives
- Coriander
- Dill
- Parsley
- Salad burnet
- Tarragon

My favourite is tarragon with peeled and finely chopped cucumbers.

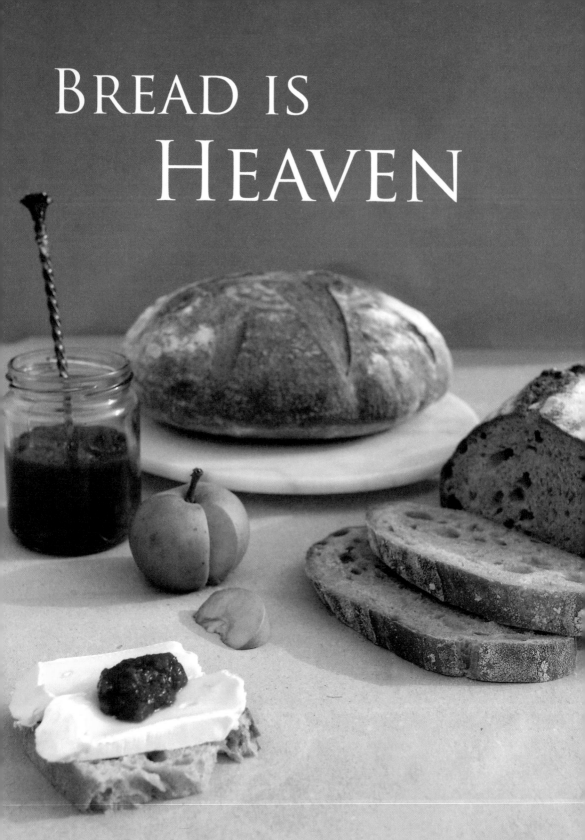

BREAD IS
HEAVEN

I think there is too much mystery made of how to bake bread. It doesn't need to be time consuming or difficult. I show you how to bake brilliant bread with the latest easy techniques and also how to make sourdough simply. When you start to make your own bread you won't want to buy it from the shops anymore.

Please use flour from local mills and not just mass-produced supermarket flours. Not only will you support a local business, you'll experience some great new tastes and textures.

All these breads freeze well. This means that you can use your time and energy very efficiently by baking in bulk. To freeze bread, either make or cut the loaves into sizes that will last you 2 or 3 days. Make sure you allow them to properly cool, then seal well in freezer bags. The freezing process does make the loaf slightly drier and this effect will increase over time. Bread will keep well for 2-3 months, after this you will begin to notice deterioration in its quality.

Note on quantities: The metric measurements are precise. For accuracy, I weigh my water: 1ml water weighs 1 gram. The conversions to cups of flour are approximate because of different densities of flours and how they pack down. Similarly, the conversions to cups of liquid are approximate too.

ROTI

Roti are my most favourite unleavened bread. Moist and rustic, they are elemental food made with the simplest of ingredients. They give you the opportunity to eat with just your hands so you're literally in touch with your food. They are the perfect partner to lentils, chicken and the red meats alike.

I gained my love of these when they were cooked by Indian and South Asian friends when I was about 6 years old. To watch the ladies of the house produce these was fascinating as they rolled them in mid-air like pizza makers in Italy. I've never acquired that degree of skill and so use a rolling pin or special velan to make the breads.

This makes a dozen roti of about 15cm (6in) in diameter.

500g (4 cups) plain flour (white or very well-sieved wholemeal or a mix of the two, or medium chapatti flour)
Water, about 350ml (1½ cups)
Pinch of salt

Optional
50-75ml/3-5tbsp vegetable oil gives a flakier result

You'll need a flat griddle, heavy based frying pan or tava to cook these on.

Mix the flour and salt together. Pour over enough water (and all the oil if using) so that you have a soft dough.

Knead the dough for 5-10 minutes by hand until it is smooth and elastic. When you press it with a finger, it should spring back. If using a machine, check the consistency every couple of minutes.

Make the dough into a ball, wrap in cling film and rest for at least 30 minutes.

Divide the dough into approximately 75g (2-3oz) portions.

Roll each portion into a ball. Use a little flour to stop things sticking and then roll out into a rough disc about 15cm (6in) in diameter and 2mm (1/10in) thick.

If you have an assistant available, they can divide and roll the dough to build up a little stock of them. Then you can start to cook, and your assistant can try to keep up. This is obviously a quicker method and you need less space to store uncooked roti. If you do not have an assistant, rest them on a floured worktop, covered by another tea towel so they do not stick or dry out.

Pre-heat your pan to very hot. You will not need any oil. Put a roti on the pan, and leave for a few seconds. Then press all over.

As you cook, you may need to adjust the heat under your pan to get the optimum result. I normally start off at maximum heat and then turn to medium after I've cooked 2 or 3 roti.

You should see bubbles forming in the dough and then brown and blacken. This will take about a minute depending on the heat. Check by turning the roti over. When you are happy with the first side, flip and cook the other side, press down all over to help it cook through. It usually takes less time to cook the second side, about 30 seconds.

The ideal cooked roti is still flexible (not crisp), and covered in brown/black raised bubbles. If you tear it, you should see the layers you've created with good kneading and rolling.

Once the roti is cooked you can just place it in a folded over tea towel and cover it over. This will keep it moist and supple.

ROTI VARIATIONS

Occasionally, I'll add something else to the roti mix. Cumin seeds, chopped fresh coriander or crushed chillies all work well. Gram flour (from chick peas) can be substituted for some of the wheat flour.

The cooked roti also make great wraps.

SOURDOUGH BREAD

You will have heard of breads called sourdough, pain au levain or sauerteig. Breads made with yeasts that naturally occur on flour have great advantages. Lots of people say they taste better and have a more satisfying texture. They also keep longer than commercially produced bread. Many people with food allergies or intolerances get on much better with naturally leavened bread.

Using natural leaven means you can control precisely what goes into your bread. All you need is flour, water and salt. No additives necessary. I think these breads are the epitome of The Permaculture Kitchen approach.

What happens is like alchemy. You'll give the yeasts the optimum conditions to multiply and grow. In turn, they'll feed on the sugars in the flour to produce alcohol, acids, heat and carbon dioxide.

The carbon dioxide makes the dough rise (it levers it up – hence 'leaven' which comes from the French verb *lever* to raise).

The acids add ample flavour. Lactic acid gives a slightly smooth, yoghurty quality; acetic acid gives the sour taste. The alcohol produced is much less than by brewer's yeasts and is of no consequence in bread making.

To get started you need a starter.

SOURDOUGH STARTER

You'll need clean water that's not heavily chlorinated. Depending on where you live, tap water may be fine, it's what I use. However, if your water is heavily chlorinated, then this additive is designed to stop things like yeast growing. In which case, a water filter would be a good investment, if not, use bottled natural, still spring water or used boiled and cooled water. Once you have the starter active, the chlorinated water should not be an issue.

The process takes a few days to get going, but you only need a couple of minutes each day. Once your starter is established, you can get into a little routine to feed it only when you need to bake.

This method makes a starter which has equal amounts of flour and water, great for everyday bread making and easy to remember. Bakers call this a 100% hydration starter.

METHOD

You need a coverable container ½ to 1 litre (2-4 cups).

Days 1-3
In your container mix to a paste:

3 level tbsp (30g) organic, stoneground rye or spelt flour
3 level tbsp (30g) organic strong white flour
4tbsp (60g) (2oz) water at room temperature (about 20°C/68°F)

Cover and leave in a place that's consistently warm (about 20-25°C/68-77°F). Any colder means it will be difficult to get things going.

Check every day for signs of bubbles at the sides and on the surface. After 2-3 days you should begin to see signs of life. The starter may smell mildly sweet. If it does, you'll feed the starter. If not, throw it away and try again.

Day 2 or 3
If you have signs of life, add to the mix:

3 level tbsp (30g) organic, stoneground rye or spelt flour
3 level tbsp (30g) organic strong white flour
4tbsp (60g) water at room temperature (about 20°C/68°F)

Cover and leave in your warm place for 24 hours.

At this stage you might want to put your container inside another container that can accommodate any overspills from a highly active starter. I use a plastic mushroom box or a soup bowl.

Day 3 or 4
The mixture should be looking a little more active now. Stir, then tip out and compost half of the starter. No need to be too precise, judge by eye.

Add to the mix:

> 40g (⅓ cup) organic, stoneground rye or spelt flour
> 80g (⅔ cup) organic strong white flour
> 120g (½ cup) water at room temperature (about 20°C/68°F)

Stir to a thick paste.

Why do you throw some of the starter away?
This is to get rid of some of the flour that has been used up by the natural yeasts. It means you can add more food (flour). A lot of people have a problem with wasting ingredients. Here, they've been used not wasted and they can go on the compost heap. Later, once your starter is established, surplus starter can be used to make other things when you don't want to throw it away.

Day 4 and each day onwards
Each day your starter should be getting more active as long as the temperature is consistent. As the starter matures, you will begin to notice increasingly:

- The smell becomes a little more acidic
- More bubbles and obvious fermentation
- A definite 'rise and fall' of the starter

Compost half of the starter.

Add to the mix:

> 40g (⅓ cup) organic, stoneground rye or spelt flour
> 80g (⅔ cup) organic strong white flour
> 120g (½ cup) water at room temperature (about 20°C/68°F)

Stir to a thick paste.

By day 7

By this time, your starter should be reacting more consistently and predictably. If all has gone well, it now should be fairly robust and will tolerate less attention.

To maintain your starter

To maintain your starter you can feed (bakers call this refresh) it each day by composting half and adding an equal amount of flour and water. If you add 120g (½ cup) of flour and water, your starter will eventually come out to 480g in weight (3¾ cups). This will be plenty to make 2-4 loaves with enough left over to act as a 'mother' for more starter.

If you do not want to bake, you can keep your starter in a cooler place for quite a few days without feeding it. I've left one out for a week and longer without feed and it revitalised after 2 or 3 feeds.

You can also store your starter in the fridge for a couple of weeks or so. It'll probably separate out into a floury sludge with some brown water on top. Tip away the brown water and half of the sludge and then refresh as normal.

In both cases, when you want to bake again, give the starter a refresh morning and late evening for two days so that it gets its vigour back.

When is the starter ready for baking?

It is ready for baking when it's near its maximum rise and before it falls back. You'll get to know how quickly it reacts in different temperatures: it can take from 4 to 8 hours or more. Another way of testing is to drop a teaspoonful into a glass of room temperature water. If the blob of starter floats, it's ready. In truth, you can use much younger starters too. You'll find out how your starter reacts the more you bake.

Changing the flour type

One final point. You can change the type of starter once it's established. This is a recipe for mixed rye or spelt and white starter. This is what I use for my standard day-to-day bread. If you want an all white starter, just refresh with the total amount of flour from strong white. If you want a rye starter, use all rye. Obviously, by the third refresh the quantity of the 'unwanted' flour in the starter will be less than 10% which is negligible.

BASIC SOURDOUGH BREAD

It's very easy to make sourdough bread once you have the hang of the slower rhythm and longer times involved to ferment the dough. This is the method I use for my everyday bread.

The amount of water is low enough so that the dough is relatively easy for you to handle. It will start off sticky and improve as the dough 'develops'. So please don't add lots more flour. You'll find it much better if you work with wet hands or oil your hands and the work surface.

This quantity of dough will make 2 large loaves. You can divide it up into smaller quantities or scale the recipe up or down.

200g (¾ cup + 1½tbsp) active starter, made with equal weights of flour and water (see page 140 for how to make it)
575ml (2½ cups) warm water
900g (7 cups) strong white flour
100g (¾ cup) spelt or strong wholemeal flour (or you can just use all white)
20g (2tbsp) sea salt, finely ground, dissolved in 50ml (3tbsp) boiling water

Pour the starter and water in a bowl and mix. Add the flour and mix until all the grains of flour are wet. I use a dough scraper to help me do this. A big spoon or your hands will both work well. You should now have a sticky, shaggy mass.

Leave for 20-30 minutes.

Add the salt and water and mix well so the salt is well distributed.

Cover with oiled plastic and leave for 1hr.

Gently spread the dough out into a rectangle about 30 x 40cm (12 x 16in), with the 30cm (12in) side on the top. Fold the top third of the dough down onto the rest and press the sides down. Fold the bottom piece of dough up to the top and press down the sides. You've just made one letter fold.

Turn the dough through 90 degrees and spread out again gently into a rectangle. The dough will be developing some strength and so you'll probably not be able to make the rectangle quite so big. Fold the top third down and seal the edges. Fold the bottom up over this and seal the edges.*

Wash the bowl and dry to get rid of dough and flour bits. Then oil it sparingly so the dough does not stick when you return it.

Gently shape the dough into a neat round and place back in the oiled bowl, cover with some oiled plastic.

This is your first folding. Leave for one hour in a warm place.

Fold again twice as before. This is your second folding. Cover with oiled plastic and leave for 1hr in a warm place. Do the same again a third time. This is your third folding.

As you fold your dough, it should change in feel from a shaggy mass, to putty-like, to resilient and elastic. You should be able to see and feel bubbles. If, after some practice, it's not strengthening enough, give it some more folds on one or more goes. Eventually the dough will be so springy and resilient and you'll not be able to fold it as easily: it tells you when it's had enough.

Then divide the dough in two and roughly pat out into a rectangle, round or oval depending on what you want the final shape of the loaf to be – long, round or batard.

Leave to rest for 30 minutes covered in oiled plastic.

Mould the dough into your final shapes and settle in proving baskets/bannetons or onto baking parchment and cover with oiled plastic and a tea towel. If you're using proving baskets/bannetons make sure that they and the tops of the loaves are well floured with either rye or rice flour. These flours will help prevent your dough from sticking. Normal flour tends to absorb more water and is much more likely to stick.

* There is a video on my website which helps to show you how to make the folds.

Allow to prove for 1½ to 4 hours. The time depends on the temperature. When the loaf is first made, the dough is very resilient. Pressed with a finger, it will push back and fill the dent.

This tests whether the gases produced by the fermenting yeast still have enough power to make the bread rise. The longer you prove the less pronounced this effect is. Ideally, you will pop the loaf in the oven before the dough ceases to push back. You'll learn to judge the timing the more you bake. With sourdough you will not get the dramatic 'doubling in size' you see in some other yeasted bread recipes. Look for a 25-50% increase.

About 45-60 minutes before you bake, preheat your oven to its highest setting. I bake on a granite stone which gives good heat to the bottom of the loaves and a good crust and rise. You can also use ceramic tiles, pizza stones or preheated oven trays.

If possible, put a tray of boiling water below where the bread will bake 10-15 minutes before you start baking to create steam.

When the loaves are proved, slash the tops. This gives the dough a weak place to split and prevents the loaf bursting in other places as it expands and 'springs' in the oven.

Place the loaves in the oven and turn it to 230°C (450°F). Bake for 15 minutes.

Take out the water tray and turn down the heat to 200°C (390°F) and bake for another 30 minutes until it's cooked right through. I tend to bake my loaves for 50 minutes so the crust crackles when it comes out of the oven. If you don't like such a robust crust, cook the bread for 40 minutes or so.

Take the bread out of the oven and allow to cool on a rack. If you like a hard crust, leave it uncovered until it's cool. If not, put a clean tea towel over the bread as this will ensure a softer crust.

BASIC YEASTED WHITE LOAF

This recipe will give you an excellent white loaf with the minimum of dough handling. It's a minimal-knead loaf rather than 'no-knead' based on a technique by Dan Lepard.

The first recipe makes a large loaf of about 1kg (2lbs). You can cook it in a 1kg (2lbs) loaf tin, or shape it into rolls, boule(s) or batard(s). You can scale the ingredients up or down. You will also need a large bowl (about 2 litres/quarts capacity or more) to mix and knead the dough in.

1tsp sugar
17g (2tbsp) active yeast
(1 x 7g/2tsp sachet Easy Bake yeast)
470ml (2 cups) warm water
(150ml (10tbsp) boiling with 320ml (1⅓ cups) cold)
730g (5¾ cups) strong white bread flour
12g (1tbsp rounded) salt

If you use dried active yeast: dissolve the sugar in a small jug or bowl with 150g (10tbsp) of the water. Sprinkle on the yeast and whisk thoroughly. Leave in a warm place for about 15 minutes until the liquid is frothy on top. Add the yeasty liquid to the rest of the water in your big bowl. Sprinkle over your flour and salt.

If you want to use easy bake yeast: simply mix all the ingredients together. Put the water in first, as this prevents the flour from going everywhere.

Using your hands, a large spoon, spatula or dough scraper, thoroughly mix the dough together. Make sure the ingredients are well combined and all the flour is mixed with water. The dough will be sticky and ragged. This is OK, so don't add more flour, it's not necessary. Pop the dough onto a lightly floured or oiled surface. Wash out the bowl, dry it and then spread some oil on the surface so the dough doesn't stick. Place the dough back in the bowl.

Leave the dough covered with a piece of oiled cling film for 10 minutes.

Then give the dough a quick knead for 10 seconds. I do this by imagining the dough circle is a compass face with the eight cardinal (N-E-S-W) and ordinal (NE-SE-SW-NW) points. So I call this a '10 Second Compass Knead'.

Take a bit of the dough at N and bring it in to the middle of the dough. You may find it helps to do this with a damp hand or a hand with a little vegetable oil on it to prevent sticking. Do this in turn with the cardinal points. Then do this with the ordinal points. Turn the dough over and make it look a tidy round and pop it back in the bowl and cover with the oiled plastic. Leave for another 10 minutes in a warm place.

Do the 10 Second Compass Knead two more times. You will have noticed the texture and stickiness of the dough has changed as it will continue to do.

After the third Compass Knead, leave the dough, covered for another 30 minutes.

Now you need to divide the dough into your desired sizes and shape it.* If you are making a loaf for a 1kg (2lb) loaf tin, grease the tin first. Or you can get approximately 12 x 100g (4oz) rolls or 16 x 75g (3oz) rolls from this amount of dough.

Cover with oiled plastic so it doesn't dry out. Preheat your oven to 230°C (440°F). Allow the dough to rise (prove) in a warm place until it increases by half the size. This will take 45 minutes to 1½ hours depending on the temperature and humidity. When it's first shaped, it's firm and springs back quickly if you press with a finger. You'll notice that the push back gets weaker as the gas expands the dough. Bake when there is still a little spring left. If it fails to push back, it's over proved and may flop.

When the loaf is ready, place in the oven and bake for 20 minutes. Then turn down to 200°C (390°F) and cook for another 20 minutes.

---

* There is a video on my website which helps to show you how to shape the bread.

VARIATIONS

You can add all sorts of things to the dough when mixing it to produce flavourful breads.

- 200-400g (¾-1¾ cups) of well flavoured grated cheese such as a farmhouse cheddar.
- A small handful each of dried tomatoes and pitted, sliced olives.
- A couple of teaspoons of dried herbs.
- A handful or two of sunflower seeds.
- Replace some or all of the flour with strong wholemeal or spelt flour for a more substantial loaf with a nuttier flavour.

A NOTE ABOUT YEAST

Most professional bakers use fresh yeast. For many home bakers, this often isn't available nor easy to keep over a household baking cycle. If you're not making sourdough or soda bread, this leaves using 'Dried Active' yeast or 'Easy Bake' yeast as raising agents. The 'Dried Active' yeast is just what it says and needs to be re-activated by adding to warm water with a little sugar for food. The 'Easy Bake' yeast contains additives like emulsifiers and acids to help 'improve' the dough.

A NOTE ABOUT SALT

Salt is not just for flavour. It helps to strengthen the dough so it can hold the gases that make the bread rise. It helps produce a good crust and acts as a preservative too. If you forget to put salt in bread you'll certainly notice the flavour difference.

My preference is to use about 1% of the final uncooked dough weight as salt.

PIZZA DOUGH

These doughs are really easy to produce. You can use them straight away or leave in the fridge for a few hours. Allow it to warm up to room temperature before you start using it. Sourdough pizza dough can even be used the next day. For ideas for topping your pizzas see pages 58–63.

500g (4 cups) strong white flour or Type '00' Italian flour (often sold as 'Pasta flour')
1tbsp Dried Active yeast *or* 2tsp Easy Bake/Fast Action yeast
1tsp sugar
8g (1tbsp) salt
330g (1⅓ cups) warm water
2-3tbsp extra virgin olive oil

Pizza dough using dried yeast

You will need a bowl of about 2 litres/quarts capacity or more to make this.

Follow the instructions for the basic white loaf (page 147), up to and including the 30 minute rest. Your dough is now ready for shaping and topping.

200g (¾ cup + 1½tbsp) of active '100%' sourdough starter (see page 140)
230ml (1 cup) warm water
400g (3 cups) strong white flour or Type '00' Italian flour (often sold as 'Pasta flour')
I often replace 100g (¾ cup) of the white flour with wholemeal spelt flour which gives a lovely nutty flavour
9g (1tbsp) fine sea salt

Sourdough pizza dough

You will need a bowl of about 2 litres/quarts capacity or more to make this.

Add the starter and water to the bowl and mix.

Then add the flour and salt and mix the ingredients well.

Cover with some oiled plastic. If you have time, fold the dough in thirds twice after 1 and 2 hours (see page 144). After this, it will be ready to use straight away. If you don't want to use it then it can rest in the fridge for 12 hours or so. Bring it out of the fridge about an hour before you want to use it to warm up.

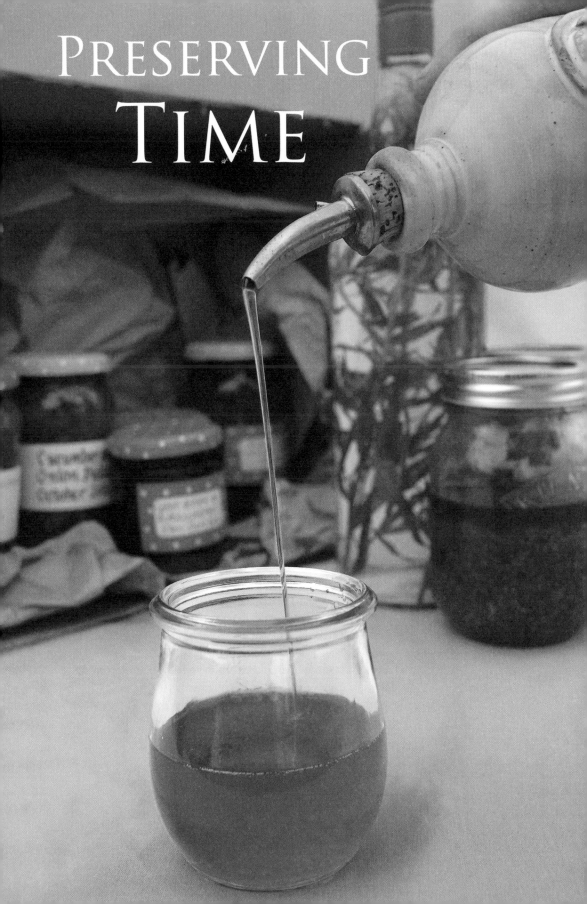

PRESERVING
TIME

The Permaculture Kitchen approach encourages you to invest in your kitchen by making things ahead. Not only do you save time, you can preserve produce that might go to waste. You'll also have some brilliant ingredients to make your food super tasty, very quickly.

Let's start off with a bang...

VEGETABLE FLAVOUR BOMB OR 'BATTUTO'

This is a useful mixture of diced or chopped vegetables, sometimes with herbs, bacon or chilli. You gently sauté the mixture of vegetables so it develops a rich, sweet and aromatic flavour (the soffrito). You can use it to start soups, casseroles, pasta sauces or as a stock cube substitute. What makes it doubly useful is that you can freeze it and just cut off what you need. It's an ideal item to make in bulk. I'm very grateful to my friend, chef Carla Tomasi in Rome, for this idea. Similar mixtures appear in the cuisines of other countries.

You can vary the texture of the battuto depending on the dish it appears in. Try a very fine battuto for soups or chunky if you are using it to cook with other vegetables as a side dish. Simply pop all the ingredients in a food processor and pulse them to the texture you desire. Or you can chop the ingredients by hand with a knife or mezzaluna.

Gently cook the vegetables so that you can extract the flavoursome juices into the oil. As they cook, they develop the blended flavours. Use a medium to low heat so that the vegetables do not brown or burn which would make the flavour harsher.

There are no real rules for quantities or content of the battuto, so experiment and see what you like. Below is a mixture to get you started. If you are vegetarian or vegan, just leave out the bacon.

METHOD

Chop the ingredients to your desired level of chunkiness.

Heat a good glug of oil or fat in your pan.

Add the vegetable/bacon mix and sauté, stirring over a medium heat until the onion starts to go translucent. Add a good pinch of sea salt, then cover the pan and reduce the heat to low. Cook for 20-30 minutes.

You can then use the battuto or freeze it. To freeze the battuto, spoon some out onto a piece of baking parchment and make into a narrow roll of about 3cm (1¼in) or so. Wrap and pop in the freezer. When you need some just cut off a slice with a serrated knife.

2 onions
5 cloves garlic
2 carrots
2 sticks celery
A small bunch parsley
A sprig of rosemary, leaves picked
75g (3oz) smoked bacon, pancetta or prosciutto or similar
Olive oil, lard or bacon fat
Pinch sea salt

VARIATIONS

Add whatever vegetables or herbs you like to the battuto. Fennel, chilli, thyme and summer savory would all be good.

You can vary the relative quantity of the individual vegetables depending on your preference or on what you have available.

The mixture will also store well in a jar in the fridge if you keep the surface covered with oil.

HERB PRESERVES

You can put quick tasty meals together with some jars of preserved herbs stashed in your fridge or freezer.

If you grow your own, this is a handy way of using up herbs in a glut or ones that are about to go to seed (to bolt). If you see a bargain in the market or get a veg box and cannot use all the herbs provided, this ensures you don't waste what you've paid for.

This method can be applied to just about any herb you like. You can add other ingredients to the basic mixture to make delectable variations.

The herb is preserved partly because it is covered in the oil which protects it from the air so that bacteria does not breed. The lemon juice or vinegar and salt also have a preservative effect. You can store this preserve in the fridge for a good six months, as long as you keep a topping of oil over the paste. If you forget to do this, the surface will soon become mouldy.

I've set out the ingredients per 100g (4oz) of herb but you can scale the recipe depending on the quantity you have. Feel free to vary the proportions to taste.

A food processor will make the preparation quicker but you can also chop the ingredients by hand with a sharp knife.

You'll need some sterilised jars to store the herbs in. You can also vac pac them or pop them in freezer bags or ice cube trays and freeze.

In French these basic preparations are called *ades*: so parsley is *persillade*, rosemary is *romarinade* etc.

HERBY FAVOURITES

These fresh herbs work well with this method, either alone or in a mixture:

- Basil
- Oregano
- Parsley
- Rosemary
- Tarragon
- Thyme

METHOD

Finely chop the herbs in a food processor. Add the garlic chunks and process until the herbs and garlic are fine without being completely liquidised.

Gradually add olive oil while the processor runs until you have a loose texture to the mixture. You may have to scrape down the sides of the processor bowl periodically so that it mixes evenly.

Once you are happy with the consistency, add the lemon juice or vinegar and salt to taste. If you are storing the preserve in a jar, top off with oil and pop in the fridge. Otherwise, pack and freeze straight away.

100g (4oz) leafy herb, washed if necessary and leaves roughly picked off stalks. (You can leave in the softer stalks of herbs such as basil)
10 cloves of garlic, peeled and roughly chopped
About 100-200ml (⅓-¾ cup) olive oil (or vegetable, rape seed, groundnut)
3tbsp lemon juice (about ½ lemon) or white wine vinegar
Pinch of sea salt, finely ground, or to taste

USE & VARIATIONS

- Stir 2tbsp or so through cooked pasta. When you drain the pasta leave some cooking water in the pan to help distribute the sauce
- Mix with flash fried squid, grilled seafood and/or new potatoes
- Spread on top of grilled or baked fish
- Use as a base on toasted sourdough, ciabatta or baguettes topped with cheese, olives or other nibbles
- Add lemon zest which makes a paste similar to gremolata and is a traditional partner for osso bucco
- Add parmesan and you have a parsley pistou to use in minestrone or other soups. Add nuts for a parsley pesto
- Add anchovies for a Provençal effect
- Add breadcrumbs for a more-ish delight
- Mix with lemon zest, chopped anchovies, a hint of ground cumin and/or paprika and a handful of breadcrumbs. Use to coat a rack or shoulder of lamb when roasting. The crunch and punch of the persillade crumbs is a great counterpoint to the soft and sweet lamb

HERB & FRUIT VINEGARS

These are a great way for you to extract and store the flavour of your favourite herbs and fruits for later use. The taste of tarragon or wild strawberries in the winter is a magical experience.

They look brilliant in pretty bottles or you can just return the vinegar into the bottle you bought it in. The method is really very easy. I make my own apple cider vinegar and store this in used, cleaned wine bottles. Improvise with what you have to hand.

TARRAGON VINEGAR

500ml (2 cups) white wine vinegar
2 or 3 sprigs of fresh tarragon, washed if necessary and well dried
1 sprig of tarragon for bottle identification

Heat the vinegar in a saucepan till just warm but not boiling.

Pop the tarragon sprigs into your chosen bottle and pour over the warmed vinegar. Cap the bottle and leave it on a sunny windowsill. Shake gently every day or so and leave for 2-3 weeks.

Take out the tarragon sprigs and replace with the fresh sprig to identify the bottle or label the bottle. With some herbs you may need to strain the vinegar through muslin or a coffee filter before you re-bottle.

USES

I use this in vinaigrettes (see page 129) and mayonnaise (page 132). It partners with all kinds of green beans extremely well and also fish and chicken.

TARRAGON VINEGAR VARIATIONS

You can use any fresh herb you like with this technique. It's great for capturing the flavour of edible flowers such as lavender, pinks, nasturtiums, elderflowers, primroses, violets and roses.

STRAWBERRY VINEGAR

Put the strawberries into a glass jar or bowl.

Heat the vinegar until it's hot but not boiling. Pour it over the strawberries, stir and cover with a clean cloth.

Leave on a sunny windowsill for 2-3 weeks and stir occasionally.

Strain the vinegar through muslin or a jelly bag, then run through double muslin or a coffee filter. Bottle and store in a dark place.

500ml (2 cups) red wine vinegar
375g (14oz) strawberries, hulled, cleaned if necessary and lightly mashed or chopped

VARIATIONS

This is brilliant made with tiny wild strawberries. I keep a jar of vinegar to hand and pop any small strawberries I do not use in this through the summer months, stirring and crushing occasionally. Then this can be strained and filtered as normal.

You can use other fruits, such as red, black or white currants too.

Perfect with vegetable and fruit salads and meats, this produces a great looking vinegar too. It's a good way of using fruit that is less than perfect

CHILLI OIL

This is a wonderfully fiery and versatile condiment.

It is possible to add other spices, herbs and aromatics to this oil but I have always found that they are swamped by the flavour of the chilli.

This will make about 1 litre (1 quart) of oil. Just scale the ingredients for bigger or smaller quantities.

100g (4oz) fresh red chillies, destalked and chopped finely – a food processor is the least risky and potentially least painful way of doing this
or
100g (4oz) dried chillies chopped or as flakes

1 litre (1 quart) of olive, groundnut or rape seed oil.

There is no point in using expensive extra virgin olive oil for example, as its flavour will be masked by the chilli.

What you do is heat the chillies in the oil. The chemical that gives chilli its heat (capsaicin) is soluble in oil and so will transfer into it and impart flavour. You do not want to fry the chillies because this will alter the flavour. So, ideally you'll need a cook's thermometer to monitor the temperature.

Save the bottle(s) for your finished oil and return the lid(s) to stop contaminants getting in.

Put the chillies and oil in a pan over a moderate heat until the oil reaches 120°C (250°F). Then simmer for 15 minutes at this temperature. Keep a close eye on this, especially if your simmer setting is not very low. You may need to take the pan off the heat periodically to help you maintain the temperature.

If you've not got a thermometer, you are looking for the oil to become warm and start to move gently. It should not bubble or smoke.

Once the 15 minutes simmering is up allow the mixture to cool in the pan. The chillies will continue to infuse in the oil. Cover the pan to keep out contaminants.

Filter the chillies from the oil using a fine sieve, muslin, jelly bag or similar.

Then pour the oil into your chosen bottles and label them. I find it's very helpful to have an oil pourer or spout fitted to the bottle. This will help you control the amount you use much more precisely.

WHERE TO USE

You can use it anywhere you'd like to impart some flavour and heat. But here are some of my favourites:

- On top of pizzas, crostini and bruschetta
- As part of the oil for frying veg for pasta sauces
- As part of the oil for stir fries and noodle soups
- As a garnish on curries, soups, stews and casseroles

TIPS

As with other brassicas, you can eat radish leaves as a salad or cooked veg

In The Permaculture Kitchen you'll do your best to get the most from the ingredients you grow, forage or buy. Here are a few extra tips I want to pass on that will help you achieve this.

MAKE THE MOST OF HERBS & VEGETABLES

Asparagus

You need to break off the woody stems at the base of asparagus to eat them. Save these in the fridge or freezer and use them to flavour stocks.

Beetroot

Beetroot is in the same family as spinach and chard. The leaves are edible, so use small ones in salads. You can use the bigger ones as you would chard; steam, sauté or boil.

Broad beans

You can make old broad beans and/or shelled broad bean pods into a silky wine. For a 5 litre / 1 gallon demi-john, boil up 2kg (4½lb) of them in 2 litres/quarts of water for 1 hour and strain. This will extract the flavour for you. Then add sugar and continue with your normal wine method. If you need to build up your pods collection, store the empty pods in the freezer until you have enough to make into wine.

The pods make a lovely purée. Boil them until tender, then use a mouli (or food processor and sieve) to purée the pods. Flavour with butter and cream, add fresh dill or tarragon and season to taste.

For a fun snack coat medium sized pods in seasoned flour and deep fry them. Eat with dipping sauces.

Broccoli

I cry when I see TV cooks take off the florets and bin the stems. The stems are really just as edible and can be used in exactly the same way.

You can also eat the leaves from broccoli and purple sprouting broccoli (in fact all the brassicas). Experiment and see what you like, some are more peppery or bitter than others: the younger ones usually less so than the older. Use them just as you would any other green vegetable.

Cabbage

It's OK to use the outer leaves as long as they're not too munched by slugs/snails etc. Give them a good wash and shred them, then add in the last few minutes when you cook soups and casseroles. They are a great match with ham, lentil and chicken soups.

The cabbage leaves also have huge flavour and crunch when you deep fry or stir fry them as part of Chinese or Indian meals. Partner with garlic, ginger and mustard seeds.

Use the stalks the same as the leaves – chunks in stews and casseroles. Chop them or finely slice to use raw, for example, in a slaw.

Carrot

You can make pesto with the young leaves of carrots. It has a wonderful savoury taste and is easy to make. You can also use the leaves as a vegetable. If you would like a natural dye-stuff, carrot leaves give a yellow-green colour, as will other umbellifers.

CARROT GROWING TIPS

If you've cut off the top of a carrot, you can replant it and new shoots will grow over winter for you to crop (with or without blanching them in the dark).

Cauliflower

Treat florets, stalks and leaves in a similar way to broccoli. Cauliflower is especially good in soups with blue cheese, nuts and red garnishes like chilli and paprika.

CARROT TOP PESTO

Here are quantities for 100g (4oz) of carrot tops. Feel free to change the ratio of the ingredients to suit your preference and what you have to hand. Scale the recipe according to how many carrot tops you want to use.

100g (4oz) young carrot tops
1 clove garlic, peeled and roughly chopped
50g (2oz) whole almonds (it doesn't matter whether they are blanched or not), hazelnuts and walnuts work well
50g (2oz) parmesan or equivalent hard cheese, cut into rough dice
150ml (10tbsp) extra virgin olive oil
Salt and pepper

Wash the leaves to get rid of any mud and grit. Place them in a saucepan with the water still clinging to them and boil for 2-3 minutes until the leaves wilt. Strain in a colander and refresh with cold water to prevent them overcooking. Drain completely and squeeze out as much liquid as you can. If the tops are very young, you can leave them raw.

Dry roast the whole almonds or nuts in a heavy based pan.

Put the almonds, garlic and a small amount of the carrot leaves into a food processor. The carrot leaves help the other ingredients process well. Blitz until the almonds and garlic are finely chopped.

Add the rest of the carrot leaves and process until puréed. You'll probably need to scrape down the sides of the blender a few times to ensure even processing. Add the parmesan cheese and process until well mixed, scraping down if needed.

You can freeze the pesto in some in ice cube trays for a winter treat

While the processor runs, gradually pour in the olive oil until you have a fluid paste. Add it gradually, stopping to test consistency and scraping down the sides. It will get to a point I call 'falling over', this is when the pesto gently falls into the blades of the processor as it turns.

Season to taste.

The pesto will keep for a few days in a jar in the fridge. Just cover the top of your pesto with a layer of oil.

Celeriac

The leaf tops of celeriac are edible. Use the young, small ones raw in salads. Use the bigger leaves as a green veg or to flavour stocks or as part of your battuto (see page 152).

Celery

I try to keep the (tougher) outer stalks for stocks or flavouring things where they will 'melt'. It is best to keep the inner stalks and leaves to use raw and as garnish in salads.

You will also find that the base of a celery head will regrow and produce shoots you can harvest.

Chilli

If you've scraped the seeds and white pith from your chilli, you can save these to use in stocks. As I said before, these contain most of the heat. I like to use them to give a warm glow to chicken stocks for noodle soups.

Courgette

Not many people know the leaves and shoots of the courgette plant are also edible. They can be blanched and dressed in vinaigrette or coated in batter and deep-fried – great with mayonnaise.

Herbs

As you might have spotted in earlier recipes, you can use the stalks of the soft stalked herbs (basil, parsley, coriander, dill) chopped up in your frying base for meals or save them in the fridge or freezer. I often keep the hard stalked herbs for stocks or you can use rosemary stalks as skewers. **However, don't use bay stalks as the wood is poisonous.**

Kohl rabi

This is a brassica and so the leaves are also edible as a normal green vegetable. You can also use the small ones in salads.

Leek

While usually discarded, the green top portion is good washed and saved for stocks, casseroles and purées.

Lettuce

You can use the outer leaves to bring a deeper and sweeter flavour to vegetable stocks as long as they are not too badly slug/snail damaged.

Onion

Save the root ends of brown, red and white onions to flavour stocks. Store them in the fridge or freezer. You can use the skins to colour and flavour stocks too or as a dye-stuff.

Save the spring onion tops you don't need and use in stocks, or pop into rice for an easy onion tang, then just fish them out after.

Pea

Treat the shucked pea pods in a similar way to broad bean pods.

Fried shucked young pods are great with mayo: garlic, pea, mint or tarragon flavours combine with them really well.

Pumpkin

You can keep the seeds. Wash and dry them well and fry for a snack or garnish. They are also delicious coated with your favourite spices and oil and fried till they pop.

Radish

As with other brassicas, you can eat the leaves as a salad or cooked veg.

Spinach and Chard

Sometimes you don't want to use the ribs in a dish. So use them in soups (see the minestrone recipes which start on page 46), stews or pizzoccheri.

Swede

As with other brassicas, you can eat the leaves as a salad or cooked veg.

Sweetcorn

Husks will make a tasty stock when boiled up. Team them up with normal stock vegetables and herbs and simmer for about 40 minutes. Use 2 or 3 for each 2 litres/quarts of water. You can then strain and use the stock: this will be great as a base for the fish chowder recipe (see page 53). You can collect the husks in the freezer to build up supplies but use the same year as picked.

Tomato

Where you've cut out the core, use them in stocks to add flavour. Or roast with other tomatoes and then strain or mouli for passata/pasta sauce.

Turnip

These are also a brassica so the leaves are edible. I love them. In the garden, they store in the ground over winter and provide a great resource for quick green veg. My favourite way to use them is as a sauce for pasta with garlic, chilli, anchovies and loads of extra virgin olive oil.

AND FINALLY...

I hope what I've written has inspired you to cook sustaining and sustainable food for yourself and those you love.

To cook for people is one of the most intimate things you can do: you feed their body and their soul.

Planning ahead and using responsibly sourced and seasonal ingredients with minimum waste and faff, helps you to sustain the planet. It's less stressful and makes sense for your pocket too.

It's easy to cook a variety of great food confidently when you use some flexible basic principles. And you don't need to spend an age every day doing it either.

Above all, cooking is fun and exciting.

What's not to like?

Buon appetito!

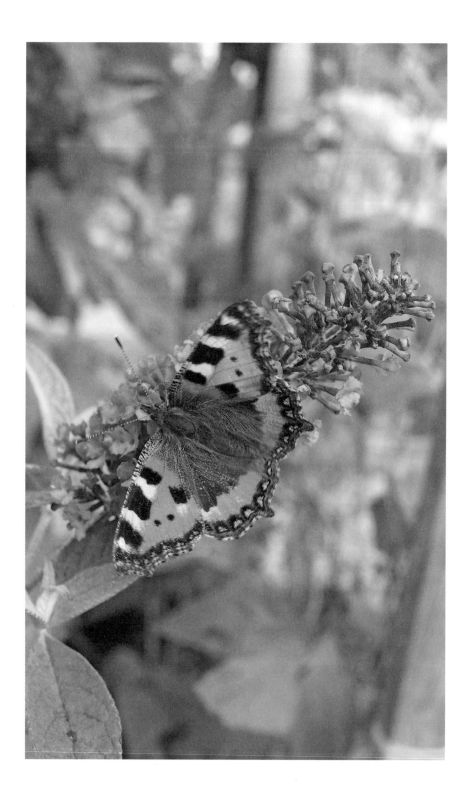

MY THANKS TO...

Maddy and Tim Harland for their confidence in me and for all their support and guidance.

Hayley for her talent and beautiful photography and design which brought this book to life.

My Twitter 'family' for their encouragement, enthusiasm, advice and knowledge. With special thanks to Carla Tomasi, for her generosity of food and knowledge, and to Helen Parkins who was always there with support and wise words.

Debs and JJ for putting up with me, especially while I wrote this book.

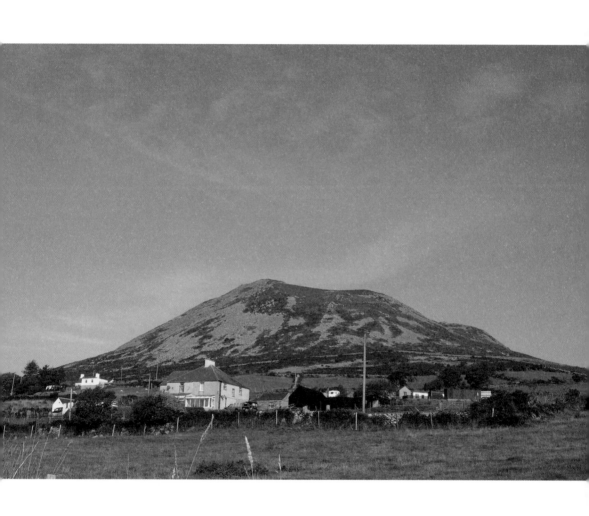

BIBLIOGRAPHY & FURTHER READING

My website, www.carllegge.com, contains more recipes and also videos of the bread folding and shaping techniques. I'll be publishing more helpful resources there, so please visit and say hello.

Larousse Gastronomique, Mandarin Paperbacks 1990.

Made in Italy: Food and Stories by Giorgio Locatelli, Fourth Estate 2006.

Vegetarian Dishes from the Middle East by Arto der Haroutunian, Century Publishing 1983.

I refer to the books above in the text and in my kitchen.

Abundance by Alys Fowler, Kyle Books 2013.
All you need to know to store and preserve your garden produce (or stuff you've bought). I confess there's stuff in there from me and a mention of *The Permaculture Kitchen*. Alys is a star.

Jamie at Home by Jamie Oliver, Michael Joseph 2007.
A seasonal tour of how to grow, cook and eat simple, no-nonsense food with great flavour.

The Flavour Thesaurus by Niki Segnit, Bloomsbury 2010.
This is an invaluable reference to flavour combinations that work. It's also a fun read.

The Pressure Cooker Cookbook by Catherine Phipps, Ebury Press 2012.
This is a modern cookbook which demystifies this indispensable piece of kit. It contains great recipes which are easy to make and well explained.

The River Cottage Cookbook by Hugh Fearnley-Whittingstall, Harper Collins 2001.
The seminal grow it, rear it, cook it, eat it book. Ethical food production and a hands-on practical guide to sustainable cooking and eating.

The Thrifty Forager by Alys Fowler, Kyle Books 2011.
A really useful reference on how to find, pick, cook and eat the free food around you.

INDEX

aïoli, 135
anchovies, 22, 131
anise, 55, 130
apples, 127
artichokes, 120-121
asparagus, 92, 161
aubergine, 25, 130

bacon, 21-22, 37, 42, 45, 97, 107, 115-116, 127, 128, 152
basil, 22, 25, 37, 38, 45, 50, 63, 67, 97, 125, 126, 135, 154, 164
battuto, 21, 24, 37, 48, 49, 152-153
bay leaves, 41, 52-53, 55, 57, 79
beans
    borlotti, 38, 50
    broad, 106, 118, 161, 165
    French, 35, 76, 97, 113, 125, 127
    haricot, 35, 50
    method of cooking dried, 52
    runner, 74, 76
beef curry, 83-84
beetroot, 25, 74, 81, 107, 161
bittercress, 60, 112, 123, 127
breads
    ciabatta, 155
    panzanella, 124
    pizza dough, 150
    roti, 138-139
    rye, 72
    salads, 124-128
    sourdough, 140-146
    white yeasted, 147-149
    wholemeal, 72
broccoli, 88-89, 162
brussels sprouts, 25, 127
butter, 32, 35-38, 41, 44, 65, 108, 110, 161
    ghee, 32, 65

cabbage, 51, 81, 85, 89, 122, 162
capers, 22, 63, 125, 127, 132, 134
capsaicin, 20, 158
capsicum (sweet pepper), 25, 71
carrots, 21, 25-26, 37, 42, 54, 69, 74, 76, 122, 123, 127, 162-163
cauliflower, 38, 71, 97, 162
cavolo nero, 127
celeriac, 42, 54, 164
celery, 21, 26, 37, 54-55, 125, 127, 164
chard, 48, 73, 74, 81, 89, 107, 161, 165
cheeses
    blue cheese, 38, 60, 162
    brie, 60
    camembert, 60
    feta, 97, 108, 118
    goat's, 45, 125, 127
    halloumi, 97, 125, 127
    mozzarella, 38, 62, 125, 127
    parmesan, 36, 51, 97, 125, 127, 128, 155, 163
    pecorino, 36, 61, 97
    ricotta, 38, 97
    taleggio, 60
chervil, 55, 135
chicken
    chermoula, 102-103
    curry, 75-77
    to portion, 75, 102
    stock, 26
chickweed, 112, 123, 127, 134
chicory, 97
chilli, 164
    chilli oil, 158-159
    trinity, 20-21
Chinese cabbage, 85
chives, 43, 45, 55, 106, 108, 120, 134, 135

chowder, 53-55, 166
cima di rapa, 85
coriander
    fresh, 69, 73, 81, 83, 88, 99, 103, 131, 139
    ground, 38, 68, 73, 75, 102
courgettes, 164
    flowers, 49, 51, 118, 120
    method of cooking, 96-97
crocslaw, 122
cucumber, 82, 135
culinary trinities, 20-21
curry, 65
    beef, 83-84
    chicken, 75-77
    dhal, 68-69
    fish, 73-74
    lamb and nettle, 78-81
    method of cooking, 66
    variations, 66-67
    vegetable, 70-72
curry paste, 70, 72

der Haroutunian, Arto, 105
dhal, 68-69
    chana, 68
    moong, 68
dill, 45, 55, 92, 99, 106, 110, 118, 135, 161, 164
dressings, salad
    garlic, rosemary and anchovy, 131
    honey, mustard and orange, 130
    mayonnaise, 132-134
    quick and simple, 130
    yoghurt, 131
dried beans, cooking procedure, 52

eggeh
    autumn and winter, 107
    omelette, 108
    potato, 110
    spring and summer, 106-107

eggs
  freeze, methods to, 105
  poached, 115
energy efficiency, 105

fennel, 29, 37, 38, 50, 54, 55,
  73, 112, 127, 153
fish
  chowder, 53-57
  curry, 73-74
  grilled salmon, 99-101
  method of cooking, 73
  pollack, 98
  salmon, 99-101
  sardines, 55
  stocks, 29
  tuna, 89, 97, 125, 127, 131
foraged greens, 60, 107, 108,
  134
frittata, 105

game, 42, 45
gammon, 42, 44, 45
garlic, 18-19, 20-21, 34,
  36-38, 42, 54, 61, 66, 69,
  73, 76, 83, 85, 88, 91,
  96-97, 101, 106, 110, 116,
  125-129, 131, 135, 155,
  162, 163, 166
ginger, 20-21, 66, 69, 70, 73,
  75, 78, 83, 84, 131, 162
goat, 78, 79, 97
green leafy vegetable, fried,
  85
griddle, 38, 92, 95-98, 102,
  103, 138
grill, 12, 90, 92, 95, 97, 98,
  155

ham, 42, 45, 48, 50, 162
herbs, 55, 164
  fresh and dried, 22
  mayonnaise, 135
  preserves, 154-155
honey, 99, 130

kaffir lime leaves, 22
kale, 50, 81, 85, 89, 107, 108
kalonji, 123
kohl rabi, 25, 50, 54, 74, 164

lamb, 78-81, 155
lardons, 22
leeks, 40-42, 165
leftovers, 10, 12, 14, 15, 24,
  31, 33, 35, 38, 42, 59, 102,
  124
lentils, 68, 75, 77, 138
lettuce, 74, 115-116, 127,
  165
  and pea soup, 44-45
lovage, 55

mackerel, 55, 99
marjoram, 55
mashua, 54
mayonnaise, 122, 131-135,
  156, 164
  aïoli, 135
  by hand, 133
  herb, 135
  ingredients, 132
  by machine, 134
  methods for making,
    132
  tartar sauce, 134
menu plan, 14
minestrone
  autumn/winter, 50-51
  ingredients, 46
  meaning, 46
  method of cooking, 49
  recipes, 46
  spring/summer, 48-49
  taste of, 46
mint raita, 82
mirepoix, 21
mushrooms, 37, 38, 70,
  90-91, 107, 142
mustard, 99, 130

nasturtium, 63, 157
  capers, 22, 63, 125, 127,
    132, 134
  flowers, 118
nectarines, 125
nettles, 38, 60, 78-79, 81,
  105, 108, 112
noodles, 87-89, 98, 159, 164
nuts, 84, 113-114, 122, 155,
  162-163

oca, 54
olives, 63, 120, 149, 155
onion, 165
  trinity, 21
orange, 83, 84, 99, 101, 123,
  130
oregano, 22, 60, 61, 62, 97,
  101, 154

painting with food, 53
pak choi, 85
pancetta, 21, 22, 37, 42, 45,
  48, 50, 53, 63, 97, 115,
  125, 127, 153
parsley, 22, 25, 26, 29, 37,
  41, 45, 48-50, 55, 67, 88,
  90, 92, 97, 106, 108, 114,
  122, 127, 134, 135,
  153-155, 164
parsnip, 25, 42, 54, 97
pasta, 12, 18-19, 27, 46,
  48-51, 87-92, 96-7, 103,
  150, 152, 155, 159, 166
peaches, 125
peas, 165
  fresh, 48
  frozen, 25, 44, 76
  soup, 44-45
permaculture
  definition, 10
  ethics, 9
  principles, 10
permaculture kitchen
  methods, 10
  principles, 10
  purpose of, 10-11
  steps, 13
  sustainability, 12
persillade, 38, 49, 51, 61, 98,
  154, 155
pesto, 38, 46, 49, 51, 61, 98,
  155, 162, 163-164
pheasant, 45, 75
pizza
  big pizzas, 59
  cheese and tomato, 62-63
  courgette, 61
  dough, 60
  foraged green, 60
pollack, 98

potato
  baked, 85
  eggeh, 110
  soup, 40-42
pressure cooker, 24, 27, 35,
  41, 52, 68, 69
prosciutto, 37, 63, 153
pumpkin, 38, 54, 71, 76,
  122, 127, 165
purple sprouting broccoli,
  88-89, 162

rabbit, 34, 35, 45, 75
radicchio, 48, 127
radish, 71, 97, 112, 120, 122,
  125, 160, 165
rice
  arborio, 36
  basmati, 31, 32, 72, 76, 79
  carnaroli, 36
  paella, 34-35
  pilaf, 32-33, 76
  recipe, 31
  risotto, 31, 36-38
rosemary, 22, 38, 43, 131,
  153, 154, 164

salad
  artichokes, 120-121
  bean, courgette feta and
    mint, 118
  blanched bean and nut,
    113-114
  bread, 124-128
  burnet, 135
  chickweed, carrot and
    kalonji, 123
  crocslaw, 122
  dressing, see dressings, salad
  lettuce, potato and bacon,
    115-116
  vinaigrette, 129
salmon, grilled
  marinades and coatings,
    101
  method of cooking, 100
  recipes, 99
salt
  in bread, 128, 149
  in stocks, 24

sardines, 55
seafood, 33-38, 55, 155
shallots, 44, 70, 134
shellfish, 55
Sicilian arancini, 38
smallage (wild celery), 55
soups
  fish, 53-57
  leek and potato, 40-43
  lettuce and peas, 44-45
  minestrone, 46-52
spices, 31, 33, 38, 55, 65-67,
  69, 70, 73, 75-77, 79, 123,
  128, 158, 165
spinach, 51, 74, 78, 79, 81,
  107, 108, 134, 161, 165
spring onions, 44, 61, 68, 82,
  92, 97, 101, 110, 165
squashes, 18, 54, 71, 76, 127,
  128, 130
stocks, 24
  chicken, 26-27
  fish, 29
  home-made cubes, 24
  vegetable, 25
strawberries, 125, 156, 157
sustainability, permaculture
  kitchen, 12
swede, 50, 166
sweetcorn, 166

tarragon, vinegar, 156-157
tartar sauce, 134
thyme, 22, 38, 43, 55, 97,
  106, 127, 153, 154
toast, 87, 89, 91
tomatoes, 90-91, 166
  fresh, 17, 20, 34, 50, 57,
    66, 68, 75, 78, 79
  tinned, 20, 34, 59, 62
tomato sauce
  ingredients, 18
  method of cooking, 18-19
  variations, 20
tortilla, 105
tuna, 89, 97, 125, 127, 131
turnip, 166
  tops, 74, 81, 85

vinaigrette, 112, 122, 128,

129, 156, 164
vinegars
  herb and fruit, 156
  strawberry, 157
  tarragon, 156-157

watercress, 123, 134
wine
  red, 37, 50, 96, 115, 124,
    125, 157
  white, 29, 36-37, 120, 129,
    131, 133, 134, 155, 156

yoghurt, 33, 45, 57, 68, 78,
  79, 81, 82, 99, 110, 131,
  140

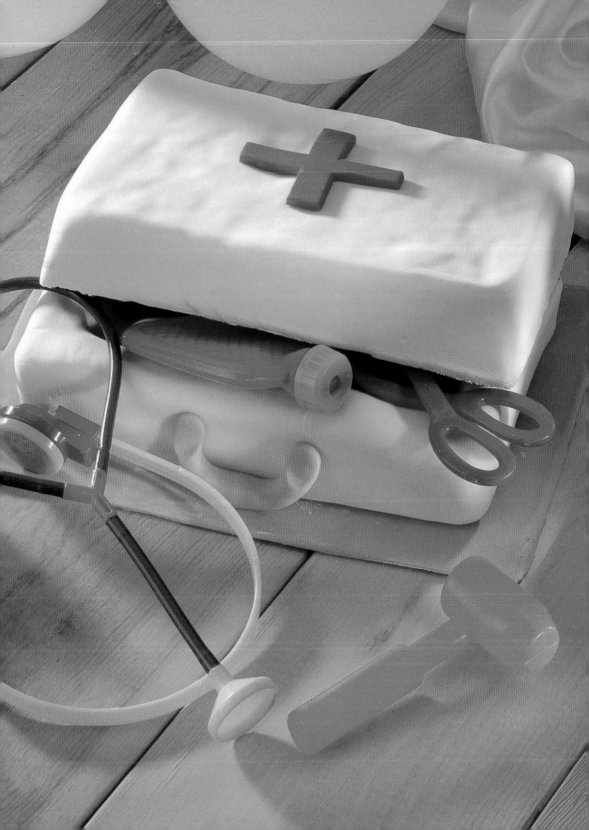

Mermaid Cake

Pretty, elegant and chocolatey! Every little girl's dream.

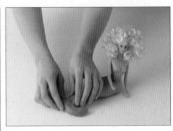

INGREDIENTS
Serves 6–8
1 quantity chocolate-flavour Quick-
Mix Sponge Cake mix
450 g/1 lb plain chocolate
25 g/1 oz/3 cups unflavoured
popcorn
450 g/1 lb/1⅓ x quantity Sugarpaste
Icing
lilac and pink food colouring
3 tbsp apricot jam, warmed and
sieved
1 egg white, lightly beaten
demerara sugar

MATERIALS AND EQUIPMENT
900 g/2 lb loaf tin
30 x 15 cm/12 x 6 inch cake board
doll, similar in dimensions to a
'Barbie' or 'Sindy' doll
small crescent-shaped cutter
small fluted round cutter
15 cm/6 inch piece of thin lilac
ribbon

Tip

For an even more chocolatey version of this cake, cut the sponge
into three horizontally and use 1
quantity chocolate-flavour Butter
Icing to spread between the layers.
Reassemble the cake and then cover
with chocolate popcorn.

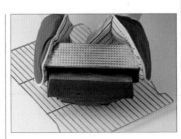

1 ▲ Preheat the oven to 180°C/350°F/
Gas 4. Grease the tin, line the base
and sides with greaseproof paper and
grease the paper. Spoon the cake
mixture into the prepared tin and
smooth the surface. Bake in the centre
of the oven for 35–40 minutes, or until
a skewer inserted into the centre of the
cake comes out clean. Leave the cake in
the tin for about 5 minutes, then turn
out on to a wire rack, peel off the lining
paper and leave to cool.

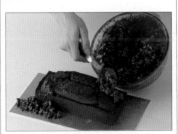

2 ▲ Turn the cake dome side up and
place on the cake board. Melt the
chocolate in a bowl placed over hot
water. Add the popcorn and stir until
evenly coated. Spoon the popcorn
around the sides of the cake and on the
cake board. Spread any remaining
melted chocolate over the top of the
cake until evenly covered. Set aside at
room temperature.

3 Cut off about one-quarter of the
sugarpaste icing. Colour the larger
piece lilac and the smaller piece pink.
Cut off about one-third of the lilac
icing, wrap this and the pink icing
separately in clear film and set aside.

4 ▲ On a work surface lightly dusted
with icing sugar, roll out the larger
portion of lilac sugarpaste icing to an
oblong shape wide enough to wrap
around the doll's legs and about 5 cm/
2 inches longer. Brush the doll from the
waist down with the apricot jam, then
wrap her in the rolled out sugarpaste
icing, lightly pinching and squeezing
it around her legs to make it stick.
Working downwards towards her feet,
pinch the end of the tail to form a fin
shape, curling the ends slightly.

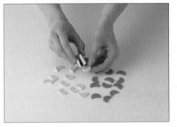

5 ▲ Position the mermaid on the
cake, moving her slightly until she
feels secure and then pressing down
firmly. Roll out the reserved lilac and
pink sugarpaste icing and use the
crescent-shaped cutter to stamp out the
scales. Cover the scales and the reserved
trimmings with clear film to prevent
them drying out. Starting at the fin end
of the tail, brush the scales with a tiny
amount of egg white and stick on to the
tail, overlapping all the time, until the
tail is completely covered.

6 Re-roll the reserved icing trimmings
and use the small fluted cutter to
stamp out a shell-shaped bra top for the
mermaid. Make indentations on the top
with the back of a knife, then stick in
place with a little extra apricot jam. Use
the ribbon to tie up the mermaid's hair.

7 Position the cake on the serving
table or large board, then scatter the
demerara sugar around the base of the
cake for the sand and add a few real
shells, if you like. Remove the doll
before serving the cake.

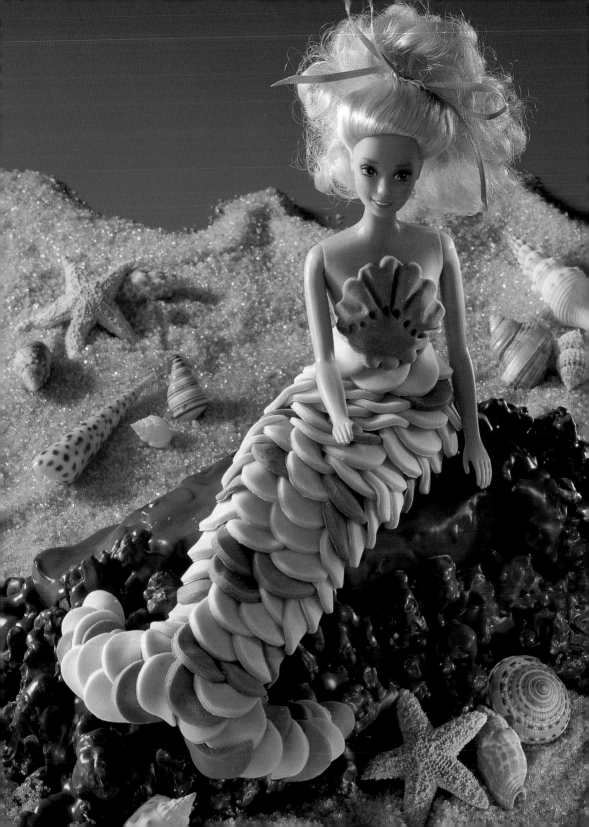

Helicopter Cake

Perfect for a party of boys or girls who are partial to helicopters.
The cake involves a little creative use of non-edible items which
must be removed before eating.

INGREDIENTS
Serves 6–8
1 quantity Quick-Mix Sponge Cake
mix
2 fan wafers
6–8 tbsp apricot jam, warmed and
sieved
450 g/12 oz/1 quantity Sugarpaste
Icing
red, blue and black food colourings
small round sweet
¼ quantity Butter Icing
2 sweets, for the headlights
2 x 15 cm/6 inch pieces of flat
liquorice
4 x 2.5 cm/1 inch pieces of liquorice
sticks
50 g/2 oz/1 cup toasted desiccated
coconut

MATERIALS AND EQUIPMENT
900 g/2 lb loaf tin
small round cutter
2 wooden skewers
wood glue
small wooden block, to raise
helicopter
18 cm/7 inch square cake board
13 cm/5 inch piece of white ribbon
piping bag fitted with a small plain
nozzle

1 Preheat the oven to 180°C/350°F/
Gas 4. Grease the tin, line with
greaseproof paper and grease the paper.
Spoon the cake mixture into the
prepared tin and smooth the surface.
Bake in the centre of the oven for 35–
40 minutes, or until a skewer inserted
into the centre of the cake comes out
clean. Turn out on to a wire rack, peel
off the lining paper and leave to cool.

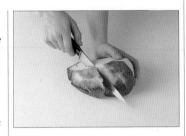

2 ▲ To shape the cake, stand it flat
side down and use a large, sharp
knife to cut it into the shape of a
teardrop. Trim the sides from top to
bottom so that the top is wider than the
bottom. Turn the cake on its side, and
cut a wedge shape out of the back part.

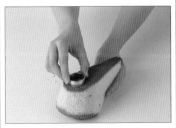

3 ▲ Invert the cake so the flat side is
uppermost. Use the cutter to stamp
out a hole for the cockpit, indenting
about 2.5 cm/1 inch. Remove the round
piece and reserve.

4 Cut a thin slice from each of the
wafers, reserve one for the tail fin
and discard the other slice. Cut each
wafer in half lengthways. Measure the
long side of one of the wafers and then
cut the wooden skewers double that
length. Glue the skewers together in the
centre to form a cross and set aside.

5 Remove a small piece of sugarpaste
icing. Take another piece of icing
about the size of an egg and colour it
deep blue. Wrap these pieces in clear
film and set aside.

6 Colour the remaining sugarpaste
icing pale blue. Remove an egg-
sized piece, wrap in clear film and set
aside. Brush the cake with apricot jam.
Roll out the pale blue sugarpaste on a
work surface lightly dusted with icing
sugar and use to cover the helicopter.
Position the covered cake on the small
block of wood on the cake board.

7 To make the propeller support,
brush the reserved piece of round
cake cut out for the pilot's cockpit with
apricot jam. Roll out the reserved pale
blue sugarpaste icing and cover the
round cake. Reserve the trimmings.
Position the propeller support on the
helicopter, halfway between the cockpit
and the tail, sticking it in place with a
spot of jam. Place the crossed skewers
on top of the propeller support and
secure them in place with a little of the
pale blue icing. Place the wafers over
the skewers, securing them underneath
with more icing. Place the small round
sweet on top.

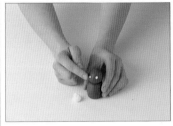

8 ▲ To make the pilot, shape the dark
blue sugarpaste icing into a small
head and body to fit into the cockpit.
Colour a little of the reserved white
icing red for the nose and mouth and
use white icing for the buttons. Stick the
details in place with a little water.
Shape some of the reserved pale blue
icing into the pilot's hat and place on
his head, securing with a little water if
necessary. Sit the pilot in his seat and tie
the ribbon scarf around his neck.

9 Colour the butter icing black and
fill the piping bag. First pipe in the
pilot's eyes, then pipe the zigzag and
straight borders around the helicopter.
Stick the headlight sweets in position
with a little of the remaining butter
icing and stick the tail fin on in the
same way. To make the landing feet,
smooth out the flat pieces of liquorice
and fold in half lengthways. Position on
the cake board, wedged in with the
liquorice sticks. Scatter the desiccated
coconut around the cake board.

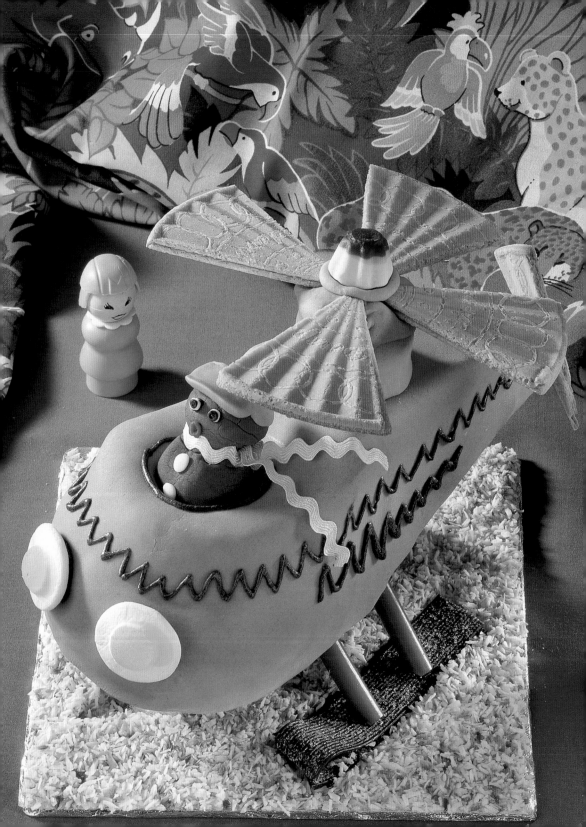

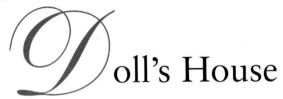

Doll's House

Little children love this cake. You can pipe their age on the door and the same number of candles can be added to the cake if you wish.

INGREDIENTS
Serves 10–12
2 x quantity Quick-mix Sponge
Cake baked in a 25 cm/10 inch
square cake tin
225 g/8 oz/⅓ quantity Butter Icing
60 ml/4 tbsp apricot jam, warmed
and sieved
450 g/1 lb marzipan
450 g/1 lb/1⅓ x quantity
Sugarpaste Icing
red, yellow, blue, black, green and
gold food colourings
115 g/4 oz/⅙ quantity Royal Icing

MATERIALS AND EQUIPMENT
30 cm/12 inch square cake board
paintbrush
greaseproof paper piping bag
No 2 writing nozzle
flower decorations

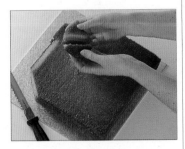

1 ▲ Split the cake and fill with butter icing. Cut 6 cm/2½ inch triangles off two corners then use these pieces to make a chimney. Shape the top of the roof. Place on the cake board and brush with apricot jam. Cover with a layer of marzipan.

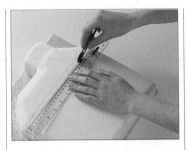

2 ▲ On a work surface dusted with icing sugar, roll out three-quarters of the sugarpaste icing and use to cover the house. Using a pastry wheel, mark the roof to look like thatch. Mark the chimney with the back of a knife to look like bricks.

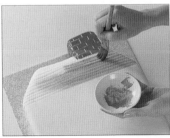

3 ▲ Paint the chimney red and the roof yellow.

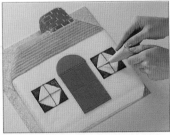

4 ▲ Mark the door 7.5 x 12 cm/3 x 4½ inches and the windows 6 cm/ 2½ inches square. Colour 25 g/1 oz/ 2 tbsp of sugarpaste icing with red food colouring, cut out and stick on the door with a little water. Colour a small piece blue, cut out and stick on for the top fanlight. Paint on the curtains with blue food colouring. Colour half the royal icing black and pipe the window frames and panes, around the door and the fanlight.

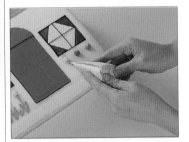

5 ▲ Colour the remaining royal icing green. Pipe the flower stems under the windows and the climber up the wall and on to the roof. Stick the flowers in place with a little icing and pipe green flower centres. Pipe the knocker, the handle and the age of the child on the door. Leave to dry for 1 hour. Paint the knocker, handle and number with gold food colouring.

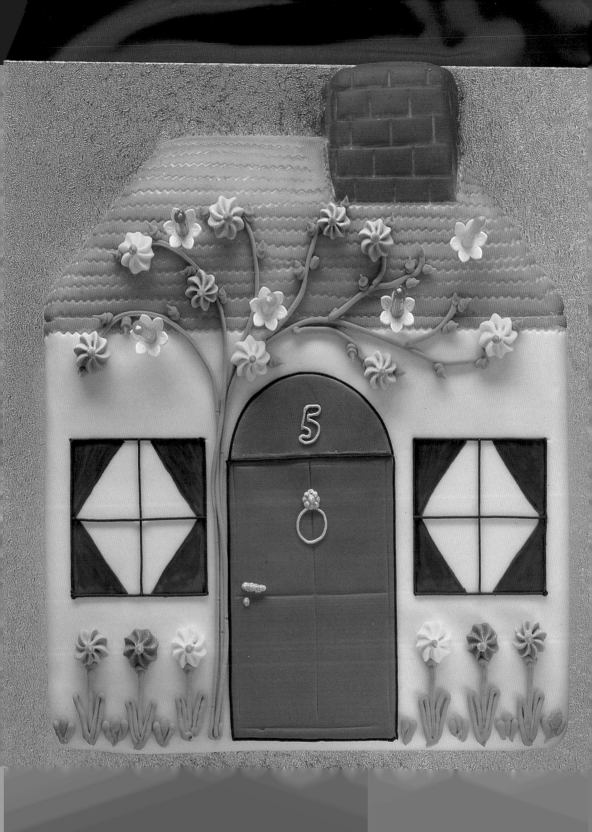

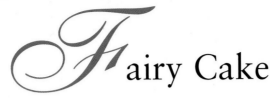airy Cake

This is one of the more advanced cakes and requires a lot of skill and patience. Allow yourself plenty of time if you are attempting the techniques for the first time.

INGREDIENTS
Serves 8–10
1 quantity Quick-mix Sponge Cake baked in a 20 cm/8 inch round cake tin
115 g/4 oz/⅓ quantity Butter Icing
45 ml/3 tbsp apricot jam, warmed and sieved
450 g/1 lb marzipan
450 g/1 lb/1⅓ x quantity Sugarpaste Icing
blue, pink, yellow and gold food colourings
115 g/4 oz/⅙ quantity Royal Icing
silver balls

MATERIALS AND EQUIPMENT
25 cm/10 inch round cake board
greaseproof paper piping bags
No 1 writing nozzle
fine paintbrush
twinkle pink sparkle lustre powder
frill cutter
small round cutter
wooden cocktail stick
cotton wool
No 7 star nozzle
silver ribbon

1 Split the cake and fill with butter icing. Place on the board and brush with apricot jam. Cover with a thin layer of marzipan. Colour most of the sugarpaste icing pale blue and roll out on a surface dusted with icing sugar to cover the cake. Leave to dry overnight. Using a template, carefully mark the position of the fairy on to the cake. As royal icing dries quickly, work only on about 2.5 cm/1 inch sections of the fairy's wings at a time. Fill a piping bag with a No 1 writing nozzle with white royal icing and carefully pipe over the outline of each wing section.

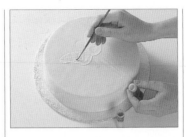

2 ▲ Pipe a second line just inside that and with a damp paintbrush, brush long strokes from the edges towards the centre, leaving more icing at the edges and fading away to a thin film near the base of the wings. Leave to dry for 1 hour. Brush with dry lustre powder (not dissolved in spirit).

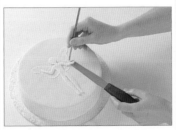

3 ▲ Colour a little sugarpaste icing flesh colour, roll and cut out the body. Lay carefully in position. Dampen a paintbrush, remove the excess water on kitchen paper and carefully brush under the arms, legs and head to stick. Round off any sharp edges by rubbing gently with a finger. Cut out the bodice and shoes from white sugarpaste and stick in place. Cut out a wand and star and leave to dry.

4 Work quickly to make the tutu, as thin sugarpaste dries quickly and will crack easily. Each frill must be made separately. Roll out a small piece of sugarpaste to 3 mm/⅛ inch thick and cut out a fluted circle with a small plain inner circle. (The depth of the frill will be governed by the size of the central hole; the smaller the central hole, the wider the frill.)

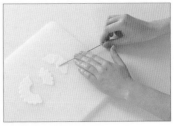

5 ▲ Cut into quarters and with a wooden cocktail stick, roll along the fluted edge to stretch it and give fullness.

6 Attach the frills to the waist with a little water. Repeat with the other layers, tucking the sides under neatly. Use a wooden cocktail stick to arrange the frills and small pieces of cotton wool to hold the folds of the skirt in place until dry. Leave to dry overnight. Brush a little lustre powder over the edge of the tutu. Paint on the hair and face, stick on the wand and star and paint the star gold. Pipe a border of royal icing round the edge of the board with a star nozzle and place a silver ball on each point. Leave to dry. Colour a little royal icing yellow and pipe over the hair. Paint with a touch of gold colouring.

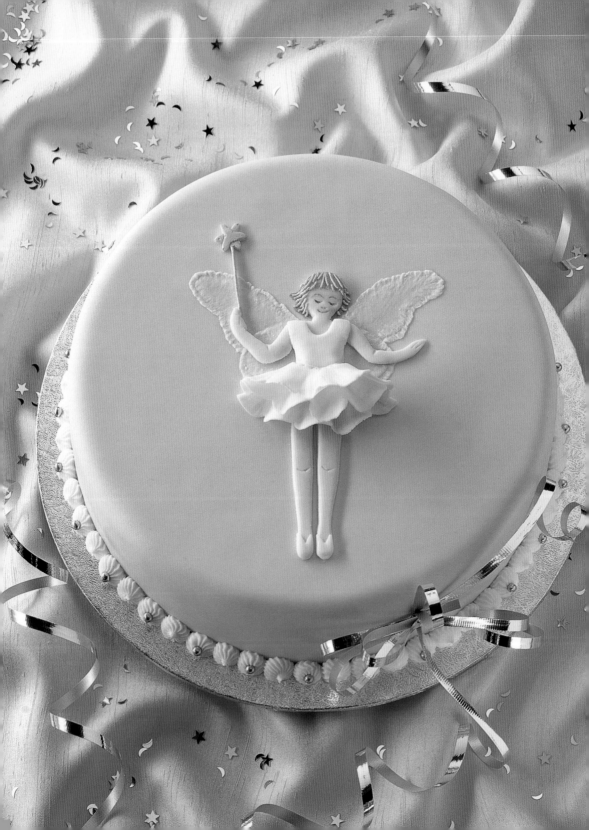

Ballerina Cake

This cake shows how you can adapt the design of the Fairy Cake to make a ballerina. The delicate pink flowers look especially pretty against the white icing background.

INGREDIENTS
Serves 8–10
1 quantity Quick-mix Sponge Cake baked in a 20 cm/8 inch round cake tin
115 g/4 oz/⅓ quantity Butter Icing
45 ml/3 tbsp apricot jam, warmed and sieved
450 g/1 lb marzipan
450 g/1 lb/1⅓ x quantity Sugarpaste Icing
pink, yellow, green and blue food colourings
115 g/4 oz/⅙ quantity Royal Icing

MATERIALS AND EQUIPMENT
25 cm/10 inch round cake board
plunger blossom cutters
frill cutter
small round cutter
wooden cocktail stick
cotton wool
greaseproof paper piping bag
No 1 writing nozzle
fine paintbrush
No 7 shell nozzle
ribbon

1 Split the cake and fill with butter icing. Place on the board and brush with apricot jam. Cover with a layer of marzipan. On a work surface dusted with icing sugar, roll out three-quarters of the sugarpaste icing and use to cover the cake. Leave to dry overnight. Divide the remaining sugarpaste icing into three: colour one flesh tones and the other two contrasting pinks for the tutu and flowers. Roll out each colour separately and cut out 12 flowers and 3 tiny flowers from the paler pink sugarpaste icing for the headdress. Leave aside to dry.

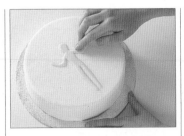

2 ▲ Make a template for the ballerina and carefully mark her position on the cake. Cut out the body from flesh coloured sugarpaste icing and stick into position with a little water. Round off the edges by rubbing gently with a finger. Cut out a bodice from the darker pink sugarpaste icing and stick in place.

3 To make the tutu, work quickly as the thin sugarpaste dries quickly and will crack. Roll out the darker pink sugarpaste icing to 3 mm/⅛ inch thick and cut out a fluted circle with a small plain inner circle.

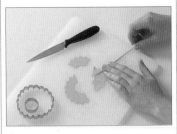

4 ▲ Cut the circle into quarters and, with a wooden cocktail stick, roll along the fluted edge to stretch it and give fullness.

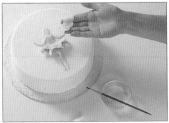

5 ▲ Attach the frills to the waist with a little water. Repeat with two more layers, using a cocktail stick to shape the frills and cotton wool to hold them in place until dry. For the final layer, use the paler pink and cover with a short dark frill, as the bodice extension. Leave to dry overnight.

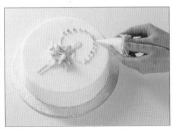

6 ▲ Attach flowers to make a hoop. Colour a little royal icing green and pipe tiny leaves in between. Paint on the face and hair. Colour a little royal icing yellow and pipe over the hair. Stick three tiny flowers in place around the head. Cut pale pink sugarpaste shoes and stick in place with water, and paint ribbons. Colour a little royal icing dark pink and pipe the flower centres on the hoop and headdress. Pipe white royal icing around the base of the cake with the shell nozzle and tie round the ribbon.

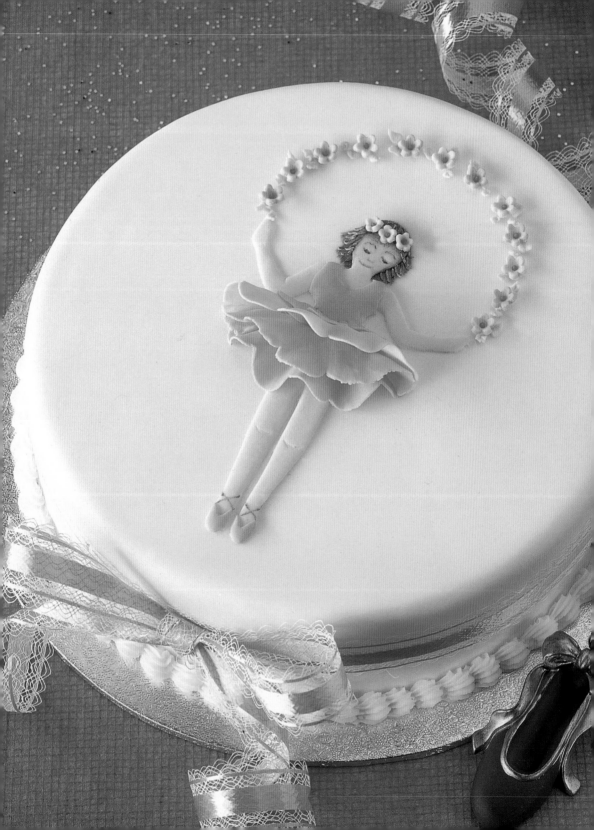

Royal Crown

The most difficult part of this cake is supporting the covered ice cream wafers with cocktail sticks while they dry in place. Plenty of royal icing can be used to smooth the joins and help to support the pieces.

INGREDIENTS
Serves 12–14
2 x quantity Quick-mix Sponge
Cake baked in a 20 cm/8 inch
round cake tin and a 15 cm/6 inch
round cake tin
175 g/6 oz/½ quantity Butter Icing
75 ml/5 tbsp apricot jam, warmed
and sieved
450 g/1 lb marzipan
575 g/1¼ lb/1⅔ x quantity
Sugarpaste Icing
red food colouring
450 g/1 lb/⅔ quantity Royal Icing
small black jelly sweets
4 ice cream fan wafers
silver balls
jewel sweets

MATERIALS AND EQUIPMENT
30 cm/12 inch square cake board
wooden cocktail sticks

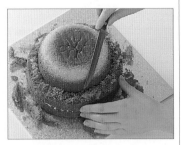

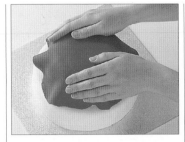

2 ▲ Colour the remaining sugarpaste icing red and use to cover the dome of the cake. Trim away the excess with a knife.

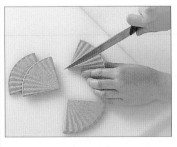

4 ▲ Cut the ice cream wafers in half with a sharp knife.

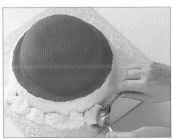

3 ▲ Spoon rough mounds of royal icing around the base of the cake and stick a black jelly sweet on each mound.

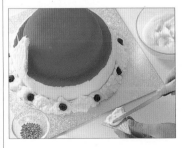

5 ▲ Spread both sides of the wafers with royal icing and stick to the cake, smoothing the icing level with the sides of the cake. Use cocktail sticks to support until dry. Put a silver ball on top of each point and jewel sweets around the sides of the crown, sticking in place with a little royal icing.

1 ▲ Split the cakes and fill with a little butter icing. Sandwich one on top of the other and place on the board. Shape the top cake into a dome. Brush with apricot jam and cover with a layer of marzipan. On a work surface dusted with icing sugar, roll out three-quarters of the sugarpaste icing and use to cover the cake.

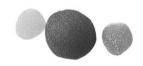

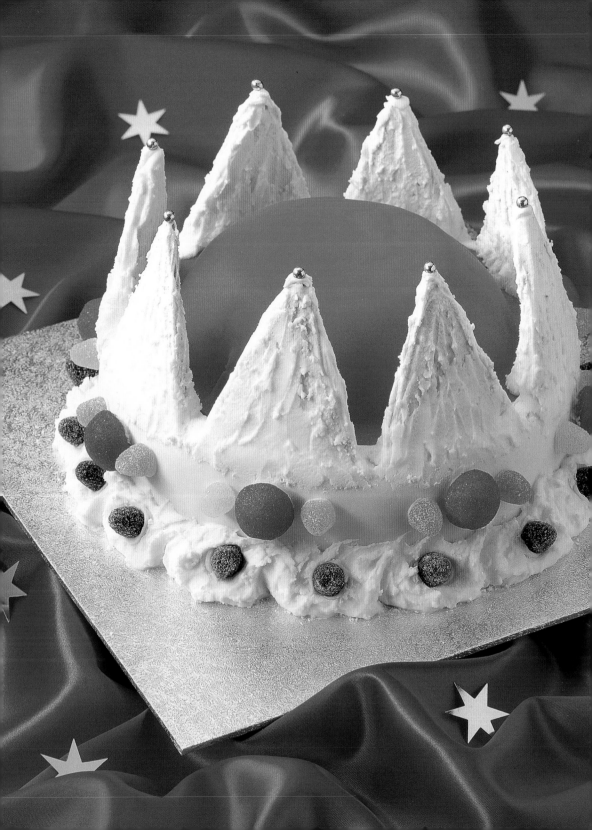

Monsters on the Moon

A great cake for little monsters!
This cake is best eaten on the day of making.

INGREDIENTS
Serves 12–15
1 quantity Quick-Mix Sponge
Cake mix
115 g/4 oz/¹⁄3 quantity Sugarpaste
Icing
edible silver glitter powder
(optional)

For the Icing
375 g/12 oz/1¹⁄4 cups plus 2 tbsp
caster sugar
2 size 3 egg whites
4 tbsp water

MATERIALS AND EQUIPMENT
ovenproof wok
various sizes of plain round cutters
30 cm/12 inch round cake board
several small monster toys

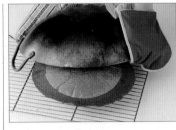

1 ▲ Preheat the oven to 180°C/350°F/
Gas 4. Grease the wok, line the base
with greaseproof paper and grease the
paper. Spoon in the cake mixture and
smooth the surface. Bake in the centre
of the oven for 35–40 minutes or until a
skewer inserted into the centre of the
cake comes out clean. Leave the cake in
the wok for about 5 minutes, then turn
out on to a wire rack, peel off the lining
paper and leave to cool completely.

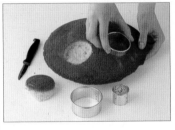

2 ▲ With the cake dome side up, use
the round cutters to cut out craters.
Press in a cutter about 2.5 cm/1 inch
deep, then remove and use a knife to
cut out the cake to make a crater.

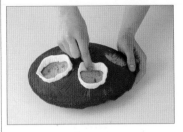

3 ▲ Pull off small pieces of the
sugarpaste icing and press them into
uneven strips which can be moulded
around the edges of the craters. Make
one of the craters especially deep by
adding an extra-wide sugarpaste strip to
make the edges higher.

4 Place the cake on the cake board.
To make the icing, place all the
ingredients in a heatproof bowl, then sit
the bowl over a saucepan of simmering
water. Beat until thick and peaky. Spoon
the icing over the cake, swirling it into the
craters and peaking it unevenly. Sprinkle
over the silver glitter powder, if using,
then position the monsters on the cake.

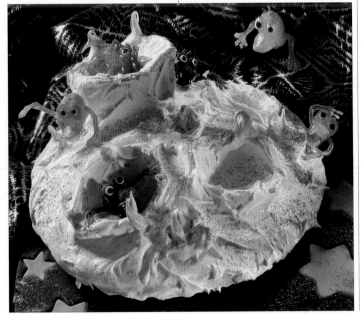

Tip

To cover the cake board, roll out
450 g/1 lb of black sugarpaste icing.
Trim the edges. Using various sizes
of star-shaped cutters, stamp out
stars from the black icing. Roll out
285 g/8 oz of yellow marzipan thinly
and use the star-shaped cutters to
stamp out replacement stars. Dust
with a little extra silver powder.

Rosette Cake

This lovely cake is actually very quick to decorate. If the icing becomes too soft, put it in the fridge to firm up. If you make a mistake, then you can always try again until you get a good finish.

INGREDIENTS
Serves 10
*1½ x quantity Quick-mix Sponge
Cake baked in a 20 cm/8 inch
square cake tin
350 g/12 oz/1 quantity Butter Icing
45 ml/3 tbsp apricot jam, warmed
and sieved
mulberry red food colouring
crystallized violets*

MATERIALS AND EQUIPMENT
*25 cm/10 inch square cake board
cake comb
piping bag
No 8 star nozzle
candles*

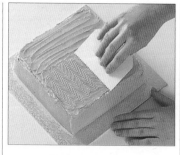

2 ▲ Using the cake comb, hold it against the cake and move it from side to side across the top to create the impression of waves.

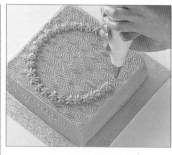

3 ▲ Put the rest of the butter icing into a piping bag fitted with a star nozzle. Mark a 15 cm/6 inch circle on the top of the cake and pipe stars around it and around the base of the cake. Place the candles and flowers in the corners.

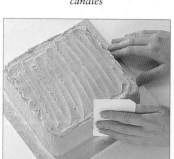

1 ▲ Split the cake and fill with a little butter icing. Place in the centre of the cake board and brush with apricot jam. Colour the remaining butter icing dark pink. Spread the top and sides with butter icing. Hold the comb against the side of the cake, resting the flat edge on the board and draw along to give straight ridges down each side.

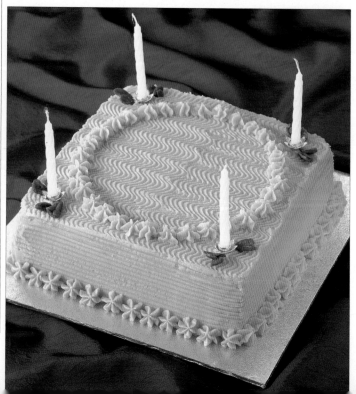

Index

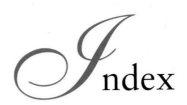

A

Almonds
  Almond and Apricot Cake, 144
  Almond and Raspberry Swiss
    Roll, 158
  Carrot and Almond Cake, 148
  Coffee Almond Flower
    Gâteau, 184
  Coffee, Peach and Almond
    Daquoise, 284
  Fruit and Nut Cake, 137
  Kugelhopf, 136
  Queen of Sheba Cake, 128
Amaretto Cake, Nectarine, 180
American frosting, 30
Angel Food cakes
  Angel Food Cake, 102
  Chocolate and Orange Angel
    Cake, 176
Animal cakes, 352–94
Anniversary cakes
  Chocolate–iced, 225
  Golden Wedding, 244
  Golden Wedding
    Heart, 230
  Heart, 296
  Silver Wedding, 246
  Sweetheart, 300
Apple Tree, 456
Apples
  Apple Crumble Cake, 98
  Cinnamon Apple Gâteau, 182
  marzipan, 62
  Spiced Apple Cake, 93
Apricots
  Almond and Apricot
    Cake, 144
  Apricot Brandy–snap
    Roulade, 290
  Banana and Apricot Chelsea
    Buns, 190–1
  Hazelnut Praline and Apricot
    Genoese, 278–9
  Lemon and Apricot
    Cake, 152
Ark, Noah's, 388
Army Tank, 445
Artist's Box and Palette, 398
Autumn Cake, 155
Autumn Passionettes, 156

B

Baking equipment, 8–9
Ballerina Cake, 500
Balloons, 470
Balloons, Birthday, 452
Bananas
  Banana and Apricot Chelsea
    Buns, 190–1
  Banana Coconut Cake, 143
  Banana Gingerbread Slices, 188
  Banana–lemon Layer
    Cake, 123
  Chocolate and Banana
    Brownies, 192
  Chocolate Banana Cake, 174
  Fig, Banana and Brazil Nut
    Teabread, 172
  marzipan, 62
Banjo Cake, 442
Barley Twist, 482
Basket of Flowers, 458
Basket, Mother's Day, 310
Basket–weave
  marzipan, 64
  piped butter icing, 68
Basket–weave Wedding
  Cake, 240
Battenberg, Mocha–hazelnut, 96
Beads, royal icing, 47
Beautiful Present Cake, 220
Bee, Bumble, 384
Beehive, 382
Bell Cake, Marzipan, 348
Birthday cakes
  Birthday Balloons, 452
  Birthday Bowl of Strawberries, 208
  Candle Cake, 454

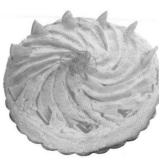

Chocolate Fruit, 210
Eighteenth, 212
Flickering Birthday
  Candle, 450
Flower, 216
Number 6, 473
Number 7, 486
Twenty–first, 214–15
  see also Animal cakes; Children's
    Party cakes; Fun and Games cakes
Black Forest Gâteau, 94
Blackberry Ring, Harvest, 318
Bluebird Bon Voyage Cake, 248
Boards, cake, 9
Boat, Sailing, 402
Bon Voyage Cake, Bluebird, 248
Bouquet, Mother's Day, 314
Box of Chocolates, 446
Box of Chocolates, Valentine's, 298
Brandy–snap Roulade,
  Apricot, 290
Brazil nuts
  Fig, Banana and Brazil Nut
    Teabread, 172
  Mocha Brazil Layer Torte, 282–3
Brownies
  Chocolate and Banana, 192
  Fudgy Glazed Chocolate, 160
  White Chocolate with Milk
    Chocolate Macadamia
    Topping, 193
Bûche de Noël, 332
Bumble Bee, 384
Bunny and Bib Cake, 206
Butter icing
  basic recipes, 28
  cake sides, 66
  cake top designs, 67
  piping, 68
Butterscotch frosting, 32

C

Cake boards, 9
Cake tins, 7, 9
  lining, 10
  quantities for different sizes, 17, 19,
    21
Cakes
  basic recipes, 12–21

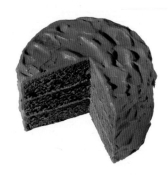

calculating quantities, 11
covering with icing, 38–42
cutting, 11
equipment, 8–9
storing, 11
testing, 11
Camping Tent, 408
Candle Cake, 454
Candle Cake, Flickering
　Birthday, 450
Car, Toy, 489
Caramel Frosted Gingerbread, 170
Cardamom Spice Cake, Pear
　and, 164
Carrots
　Autumn Passionettes, 156
　Carrot and Almond Cake, 148
　Carrot Cake, 108
　Spiced Passion Cake, 186
Cassata Siciliana, 112
Castle, Fairy, 478
Castle, Sand, 432
Cat in a Basket, 378
Cat on a Mat, sugarpaste, 54
Caterpillar, Crazy, 394
Champagne Wedding Cake, 242
Cheesecakes
　Baked Cheesecake with Fresh
　　Fruits, 116
　Chilled Grape, 118
　Luxury White Chocolate, 270–1
Chelsea Buns, Banana and
　Apricot, 190–1
Cherries
　Black Forest Gâteau, 94
　Chocolate and Fresh Cherry
　　Gâteau, 260–1
　Jewel Cake, 274
Chess Board, 414
Chest, Treasure, 430
Chestnut purée
　Bûche de Noël, 332
　Chestnut Cake, 140
　Chocolate Chestnut Roulade, 256
Children's party cakes, 450–505

Chilli peppers, marzipan, 62
Chocolate, 74
　–dipped fruit and nuts, 79
　Chocolate–iced Anniversary Cake, 225
　coating cakes, 74
　curls, 79
　cut–outs, 78
　fudge frosting, 33
　leaves, 78, 235
　marbling, 76
　melting, 73
　piping, 75
　run–outs, 76
　satin chocolate icing, 34
　shavings, 79
Chocolate cakes
　Best–ever, 100–1
　Chocolate and Banana
　　Brownies, 192
　Chocolate Banana Cake, 174
　Chocolate Cappuccino, 264–5
　Chocolate Chestnut Roulade, 256
　Chocolate and Fresh Cherry
　　Gâteau, 260–1
　Chocolate Fruit Birthday Cake, 210
　Chocolate Gâteau Terrine, 258
　Chocolate Madeira Cake, 210, 234
　Chocolate Mint–filled Cupcakes, 154
　Chocolate and Orange Angel
　　Cake, 176
　Chocolate Pecan Torte, 273
　Death by Chocolate, 268–9
　French, 267
　Fudgy Glazed Chocolate
　　Brownies, 160
　Gorgeous, 266
　Hazelnut Chocolate Meringue Torte
　　with Pears, 162
　Jazzy Chocolate Gâteau, 315
　Luxury White Chocolate
　　Cheesecake, 270–1
　Marbled Chocolate Peanut Butter
　　Cake, 194
　Mississippi Mud Cake, 132–3
　Queen of Sheba Cake, 128
　Sachertorte, 130
　Simple, 92
　Vegan Chocolate Gâteau, 151
　White Chocolate Brownies with
　　Milk Chocolate Macadamia
　　Topping, 193
　White Chocolate Mousse Strawberry
　　Cake, 262
Chocolates, Box of, 446
Chocolates, Valentine's Box of, 298
Christening cakes
　Barley Twist, 482
　Bunny and Bib, 206
　Daisy, 200
　Frills and Flowers, 202

Sampler, 204
Teddy Bear, 198
Christmas cakes
　Bûche de Noël, 332
　Christmas Cracker, 346
　Christmas Stocking, 340
　Christmas Tree, 336
　Glazed Christmas Ring, 330
　Glittering Star, 328
　Hand–painted, 344
　Marbled Cracker, 334
　Marzipan Bell, 348
　Mini, 342
　Noël, 338
Cinnamon Apple Gâteau, 182
Circus Cake, 421
Classic Wedding Cake, 236
Cloth Cake, 484
Cloth of Roses Cake, 222
Clown Cake, 422
Clown Face, 474
Clown, Happy, 428
Cobweb effect glacé icing, 70
Coconut
　Banana Coconut Cake, 143
　for cake decoration, 82
　Caramel Frosted Gingerbread, 170
Coffee
　Chocolate Cappuccino Cake, 264–5
　Coffee Almond Flower Gâteau, 184
　Coffee, Peach and Almond
　　Daquoise, 284
　Father's Day Cake, 316
Coffin, Hallowe'en, 321
Colours, 43
　flicking, 80
　linework, 80
　marbling, 52
　painting and drawing, 81
　powdered tints, 43, 81
　royal icing piped flowers, 49
　run–outs, 50
　stencils, 80
　stippling, 81
Computer Game, 440
Cooking times, 11

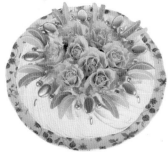

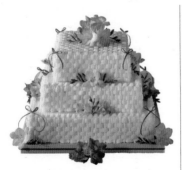

Cornelli, royal icing, 46
Cornets, Ice–cream, 433
Courgettes, Spiced Passion
    Cake, 186
Cow, Daisy, 366
Cracker Cake, Marbled, 334
Cracker, Christmas, 346
Crazy Caterpillar, 394
Crème au Beurre, 29
Crimping
    marzipan, 60
    sugarpaste, 53
Crown, Royal, 502
Cupcakes
    Chocolate Mint-filled, 154
    Decorated, 178
Curls
    chocolate, 75, 79
    ribbon, 86
Cut–outs
    chocolate, 78
    marzipan, 61
    sugarpaste, 56
Cutting cakes, 11

Daisy Christening Cake, 200
Daisy Cow, 366
Dart Board, 410
Death by Chocolate, 268–9
Decorations, bought
    edible, 82–4
    ribbons, 86–7
    stencilling, 84
    sugar–frosted flowers and
        fruit, 88–9
Diamond butter icing, 67
Dinosaur Cake, 368
Doll's House, 496
Dots, royal icing, 47
Double Heart Engagement
    Cake, 224
Drawing and painting colours, 81

Drum Cake, 444
Ducks on a Pond, 370
Dumper Truck, 462
Dundee Cake, 106

Easter cakes
    Easter Egg Nest Cake, 305
    Fruit, 308
    Simnel, 304
    Sponge, 306
Eggs, 7
Eighteenth Birthday Cake, 212
Elephant Cake, 356
Elephant, Indian, 358
Embossing
    marzipan, 60
    sugarpaste, 53
Embroidery, royal icing, 46
Engagement cakes
    Double Heart, 224
    Sweetheart, 300
Equipment
    baking, 8–9
    icing, 22–3
Exotic Celebration Gâteau, 272

Fairy Cake, 498
Fairy Castle, 478
Fan effect glacé icing, 71
Father's Day cakes
    coffee–flavoured, 316
    Jazzy Chocolate Gâteau, 315
Feather effect glacé icing, 71
Feathered spiral butter
    icing, 67
Fig, Banana and Brazil
    Nut Teabread, 172
Fire Engine, 480
Fish Cake, 360
Flickering Birthday
    Candle Cake, 450
Flicking colour
    effect, 80
Flour, sifting, 7
Flower Birthday
    Cake, 216
Flowerpot,
    Terracotta, 312
Flowers
    glacé icing marbled, 72
    made with edible decorations, 84
    marzipan, 61, 65

    royal icing piped, 49
    sugar–frosted, 88–9
    sugarpaste plunger
        blossoms, 57
Flowers, Basket of, 458
Food colourings see Colours
French Chocolate Cake, 267
Frills and Flowers Christening
    Cake, 202
Frills, sugarpaste, 58
Frog Prince, 392
Fruit
    Baked Cheesecake with Fresh
        Fruits, 116
    Chocolate Fruit Birthday
        Cake, 210
    chocolate–dipped, 79
    citrus, 82
    Exotic Celebration
        Gâteau, 272
    Fresh Fruit Genoese, 276
    Genoese Cake with Fruit and
        Cream, 124
    glacé and crystallised, 82
    marzipan, 62
    Midsummer Wedding Cake, 238–9
    Savarin with Fresh Berries, 104
    sugar–frosted, 88–9
    see also individual fruits
        e.g. Bananas
Fruit cakes
    Dundee, 106
    Easter, 308
    Flourless, 150
    Fruit and Nut, 137
    Glazed Christmas Ring, 330
    Irish Whiskey, 122
    Kugelhopf, 136
    Light, 20–1
    Rich, 18–19
    Simnel, 304
    storage, 11

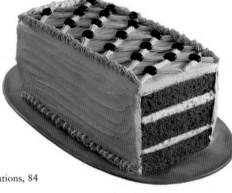

testing, 11
Fudge frosting, 33
Fudge–frosted Starry Roll, 218
Fudgy Glazed Chocolate
  Brownies, 160
Fun and Games cakes, 398–447

Gâteaux
  Black Forest, 94
  Chocolate and Fresh
    Cherry, 260–1
  Chocolate Gâteau Terrine, 258
  Cinnamon Apple, 182
  Coffee Almond Flower, 184
  Coffee, Peach and Almond
    Daquoise, 284
  Exotic Celebration, 272
  Iced Paradise Cake, 280–1
  Jazzy Chocolate, 315
  Mocha Brazil Layer Torte, 282
  Strawberry, 134
  Strawberry Cream, 291
  Tia Maria, 288–9
  Vegan Chocolate, 151
Genoese sponges
  Cinnamon Apple Gâteau, 182
  Fresh Fruit, 276
  Genoese Cake with Fruit and
    Cream, 124
  Hazelnut Praline and
    Apricot, 278–9
Ghostly Spectre, 326
Gift–wrapped Parcel, 447
Ginger Cake, Upside–down Pear
  and, 145
Gingerbread
  Banana Gingerbread Slices, 188
  Caramel Frosted, 170
  Sticky Gingerbread Loaf, 120
Glacé icing
  basic recipe, 31
  cobweb effect, 70
  fan effect, 71
  feather effect, 71
  marbled flowers and leaves, 72
  piping, 72, 73
  squiggle icing, 72
Glittering Star, 328
Golden Wedding Cake, 244
Golden Wedding Heart Cake, 230
Gooseberry Cake, 153
Grapes
  Chilled Grape Cheesecake, 118
  marzipan, 62
Greek New Year Cake, 295
Greengages, Autumn Cake, 155

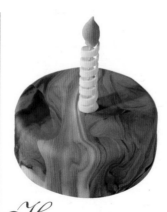

Hallowe'en cakes
  Coffin, 321
  Ghostly Spectre, 326
  Pumpkin, 322
  Pumpkin Patch, 320
  Spider's Web, 324
Happy Clown, 428
Harvest Blackberry Ring, 318
Hazelnuts
  Autumn Cake, 155
  Hazelnut Chocolate Meringue Torte
    with Pears, 162
  Hazelnut Praline and Apricot
    Genoese, 278–9
  Mocha–hazelnut Battenberg, 96
Heart Cake, Golden
  Wedding, 230
Heart Cake, Valentine's, 296
Heart Engagement Cake,
  Double, 224
Helicopter Cake, 494
Hickory Dickory Dock, 386
Honey Nut Cake,
  Spiced, 166
Horseshoe, Lucky, 228
Hot Dog Cake, 420

Ice–cream Cornets, 433
Icings
  basic recipes, 24–36
  colouring, 43
  covering cakes with, 38–42
  equipment, 22–3
  see also types of icing
    e.g. Royal
Indian Elephant, 358
Irish Whiskey Cake, 122

Jack–in–the–Box Cake, 426–7
Jazzy Chocolate Gâteau, 315
Jewel Cake, 274

Kite Cake, 476
Kugelhopf, 136
Kulich, 114

Lace curls, chocolate, 75
Ladybird Cake, 352
Leaves
  chocolate, 78, 235
  glacé icing marbled, 72
  marzipan, 61
  royal icing, 46
Lemons
  Banana–lemon Layer Cake, 123
  Lemon and Apricot Cake, 152
  Lemon Chiffon Cake, 286–7
  St Clements Marbled
    Crown, 168
Lines
  colour effects, 80
  royal icing, 47
Lining cake tins, 10
Lion Cake, 374
Liquorice Sweet Cake, 406
Lucky Horsehoe, 228

Macadamia Topping, White
  Chocolate Brownies with Milk
  Chocolate, 193
Madeira cake
  basic recipe, 16–17
  chocolate, 210, 234
  Crunchy–topped, 142
Magic Carpet Cake, 424
Magic Rabbit, 390
Map, Treasure, 471
Marbled cakes
  Chocolate Peanut Butter, 194
  St Clements Marbled Crown, 168
  Spice Cake, 99
Marbling (icing)
  chocolate, 76

glacé icing flowers and
leaves, 72
Marbled Cracker Cake, 334
sugarpaste, 52
Market Stall, 436
Marzipan, 24
basic recipe, 24
Bell Cake, 348
covering cakes for royal
icing, 39
covering cakes for sugarpaste
icing, 38
crimping, 60
cut–outs, 61
embossing, 60
modelling, 62
plaiting and weaving, 64
roses, 65
Measurements, 7
calculating servings, 11
Light Fruit Cake chart, 21
Madeira Cake chart, 17
Rich Fruit Cake chart, 19
Meringue
Coffee, Peach and Almond
Daquoise, 284
frosting, 35
Hazelnut Chocolate Meringue Torte
with Pears, 162
Midsummer Wedding Cake, 238–9
Mermaid Cake, 492
Merry-go-round Cake, 466–7
Midsummer Wedding Cake, 238–9
Mint-filled Cupcakes,
Chocolate, 154
Mississippi Mud Cake, 132–3
Mobile Phone Cake, 416
Mocha Brazil Layer Torte, 282–3
Mocha–hazelnut Battenberg, 96
Modelling
marzipan, 62
sugarpaste, 54
Monsters on the Moon, 504
Mother's Day cakes
Basket, 310
Bouquet, 314
Box of Chocolates, 298
Terracotta Flowerpot, 312
Mouse in Bed, 380
Music, Sheet of, 441

Nectarine Amaretto Cake, 180
New Year cakes
Greek, 295
Starry, 294
Noah's Ark, 388

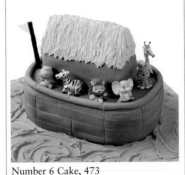

Number 6 Cake, 473
Number 7 Cake, 486
Nurse's Set, 490
Nuts
for cake decoration, 82
chocolate–dipped, 79
see also types of nut
e.g. Almonds

Oranges
Chocolate and Orange Angel
Cake, 176
St Clements Marbled Crown, 168
Orchid Wedding Cake,
Trailing, 232
Outlines, chocolate, 75
Oven temperatures, 7

Paddling Pool, 488
Painting and drawing
colours, 81
Palette, Artist's Box and, 398
Panforte, 110
Pansy Retirement Cake, 250
Pansy, royal icing piped, 49
Paradise Cake, Iced, 280–1
Parcel, Gift–wrapped, 447
Parrot, Tropical, 364
Passion cakes
Autumn Passionettes, 156
Spiced, 186
Peaches
Coffee, Peach and Almond
Daquoise, 284
Peach Swiss Roll, 126
Peanut Butter Cake, Marbled
Chocolate, 194

Pears
Hazelnut Chocolate Meringue Torte
with Pears, 162
Pear and Cardamom Spice
Cake, 164
Upside–down Pear and Ginger
Cake, 145
Pecan nuts
Autumn Cake, 155
Chocolate Pecan Torte, 273
Peepo Rabbits, 376
Peppers, marzipan, 62
Personal Stereo, 418
Petal paste, 36
Phone Cake, Mobile, 416
Pinball Machine, 438
Piping
bags, 44–5
butter icing, 68
chocolate, 75
glacé icing, 72, 73
royal icing, 27, 45, 46–50
Pirate's Hat, 472
Pistachio nuts, Spiced Honey Nut
Cake, 166
Pizza Cake, 434
Plaits, marzipan, 64
Plaques, sugarpaste, 59
Plums, Autumn Cake, 155
Plunger blossom cutters, 57
Porcupine Cake, 362
Present Cake, Beautiful, 220
Prunes, Autumn Cake, 155
Pumpkin, Hallowe'en, 322
Pumpkin Patch, Hallowe'en, 320
Puppies in Love, 372

Quantities for different tin sizes
Light fruit cakes, 21
Madeira cakes, 17
Rich fruit cakes, 19
Queen of Sheba Cake, 128

Rabbit, Magic, 390
Rabbit, sugarpaste, 54
Rabbits, Peepo, 376
Racing Circuit, 468–9
Rainbow Snake Cake, 354
Raspberry Swiss Roll, Almond
and, 158
Retirement Cakes
hexagonal, 252

Pansy, 250
Ribbons, 86
  curls, 86
  designs, 86
  insertion, 87
  loops, 86
  ovals, 86
Ridge squares, butter
  icing, 67
Ridged spiral, butter
  icing, 67
Ropes
  marzipan candy–stripe, 64
  royal icing twisted, 46
Rose Blossom Wedding
  Cake, 226
Roses
  marzipan, 65
  royal icing piped, 49
Roses Cake, Cloth of, 222
Rosette Cake, 505
Rough icing, 41
Roulades
  Apricot Brandy–
    snap, 290
  Chocolate Chestnut, 256
Royal Crown, 502
Royal icing
  basic recipes, 26
  consistencies, 27
  covering round
    cakes, 40
  covering square
    cakes, 41
  piped flowers, 49
  piped sugar pieces, 48
  piping bags, 44–5
  piping shapes, 46–7
  rough icing, 41
  run–outs, 50
Run–outs
  chocolate, 76
  royal icing, 27, 50

Sachertorte, 130
Sailing Boat, 402
St Clements Marbled Crown, 168
Sampler, Christening, 204
Sand Castle, 432
Satin chocolate icing, 34
Savarin with Fresh Berries, 104
Scrolls, royal icing, 46
Servings, calculating, 11
7 Cake, Number, 486
Shavings, chocolate, 79
Sheet of Music, 441
Shells, royal icing, 47
Shirt and Tie Cake, 404
Shortcake, Summer
    Strawberry, 185
Silver Wedding Cake, 246
Simnel Cake, 304
6 Cake, Number, 473
Snake Cake, Rainbow, 354
Snowman, sugarpaste, 54
Space ship, 412
Spice Cake, Marbled, 99
Spice Cake, Pear and
    Cardamom, 164
Spiced Apple Cake, 93
Spiced Honey Nut Cake, 166
Spiced Passion Cake, 186
Spider's Web Cake, 324
Spirals, butter icing, 67
Sponge cakes
    Carrot and Almond Cake, 148
    Chocolate and Orange Angel
      Cake, 176
    One–stage Victoria Sandwich, 146
    Quick–mix, 12
    Whisked, 13
    see also Genoese sponges
Squares, butter icing, 67
Squiggle glacé icing, 72
Star, Glittering, 328
Starry New Year Cake, 294
Stars, royal icing, 46
Stencils, 84
    colour effects, 80
Stereo, Personal, 418
Stippling colour effect, 81
Storage of cakes, 11
Strawberries
    Genoese Cake with Fruit and
      Cream, 124
    Strawberry Cream Gâteau, 291
    Strawberry Gâteau, 134
    Summer Strawberry Shortcake, 185
    White Chocolate Mousse Strawberry
      Cake, 262
Strawberries, Birthday Bowl of, 208

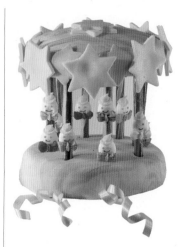

Strawberry Cake, 400
Sugar pieces, royal icing, 48
Sugar–frosted flowers and fruit, 88–9
Sugarpaste icing
  basic recipe, 25
  covering awkward shapes, 42
  covering a cake, 42
  crimping, 53
  cut–outs, 56
  embossing, 53
  frills, 58
  marbling, 52
  modelling, 54
  plaques, 59
  plunger blossoms, 57
Summer Strawberry Shortcake, 185
Sweet Cake, Liquorice, 406
Sweetheart Cake, 300
Sweets, 82
Swirls
  butter icing, 67
  royal icing, 46
Swiss rolls
  Almond and Raspberry, 158
  Apricot Brandy–snap Roulade, 290
  basic recipe, 14
  Chocolate Chestnut Roulade, 256
  Fudge–frosted Starry Roll, 218
  Peach, 126
  Whisked Sponge Cake, 13

Tank, Army, 445
Teabreads
  Banana–lemon Layer Cake, 123
  Fig, Banana and Brazil Nut
    Teabread, 172

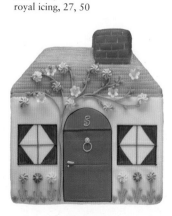

Teddy Bear Christening
    Cake, 198
Teddy bear, sugarpaste, 54
Teddy's Birthday, 385
Telephone Cake, 460
Telephone Cake, Mobile, 416
Tent, Camping, 408
Terracotta Flowerpot, 312
Terrine, Chocolate
    Gâteau, 258
Testing cakes, 11
Thermometers, oven, 7
Tia Maria Gâteau, 288–9
Tins, cake, 7, 9
    lining, 10
    quantities for different sizes, 17, 19,
    21
Tints, 43, 81
    see also Colours
Torte
    Chocolate Pecan, 273
    Hazelnut Chocolate Meringue Torte
        with Pears, 162
    Mocha Brazil Layer, 282–3
    Sachertorte, 130
Toy Car, 489
Trailing Orchid Wedding
    Cake, 232
Train Cake, 464
Treasure Chest, 430
Treasure Map, 471
Tree, Apple, 456
Trellises, royal icing, 47
Tropical Parrot, 364
Truck, Dumper, 462
Truffle Cake Mix, 15
Twenty–first Birthday
    Cake, 214–15
Twists, marzipan, 64

Upside–down Pear and Ginger
    Cake, 145

Valentine's Day cakes
    Box of Chocolates, 298
    Heart, 296
    Heart–shaped, 302
    Sweetheart, 300
Vegan Chocolate Gâteau, 151
Victoria Sandwich, One–
    stage, 146
Violets, marzipan, 61

Walnuts
    Banana–lemon Layer
        Cake, 123
    Carrot Cake, 108
Weaving, marzipan, 64
Wedding cakes
    Basket–weave, 240
    Champagne, 242
    Chocolate Leaf, 234–5
    Classic, 236
    Heart, 296
    Lucky Horseshoe, 228
    Midsummer, 238–9
    Rose Blossom, 226
    Trailing Orchid, 232
Whiskey Cake, Irish, 122

Yeast cakes
    Banana and Apricot Chelsea
        Buns, 190–1
    Kugelhopf, 136
    Kulich, 114
    Savarin with Fresh
        Berries, 104

Zigzags, royal icing, 47

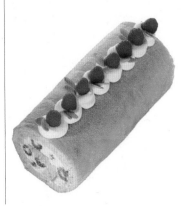

Acknowledgements

The publisher and authors would like to thank the following for supplying props
and equipment for photography: Scenics Cakes Boards, Colours Direct,
the Cloth Store, Cake Fayre, Jean Ainger, Braun and Kenwood.
Thanks also to Stork Cookery Service for the Rich Fruit Cake chart,
and Jackie Mason, Mavis Giles and Teresa Goldfinch for their help.

Enjoyed this book?

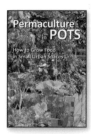
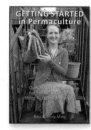
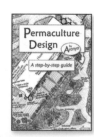
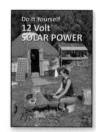
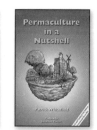

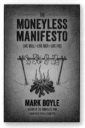
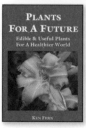
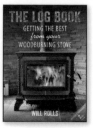
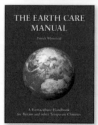
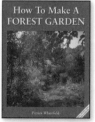

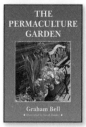
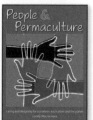
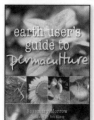
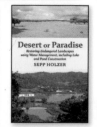
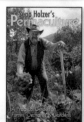

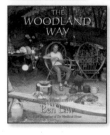
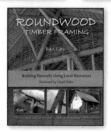
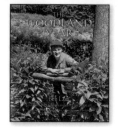
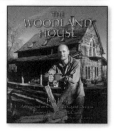

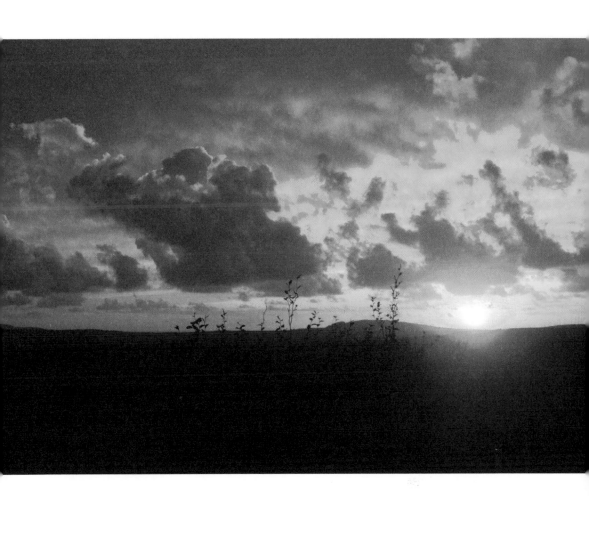